I will CURE my Parkinson's

Beyond the Prescription Pad: Navigating both Medical and Holistic treatments

By

Lisa Bradbury

*For Simon, Zachary and Jamieson who inspire
me everyday to beat this illness.*

CONTENT

PROLOGUE

Neurological disorders are medically defined as disorders that affect the brain as well as the nerves found throughout the human body and the spinal cord. Structural, biochemical or electrical abnormalities in the brain, spinal cord or other nerves can result in a range of symptoms. Examples of symptoms include paralysis, muscle weakness, poor coordination, loss of sensation, seizures, confusion, pain and altered levels of consciousness.

Examples of neurological conditions are:

- brain cancer.
- cerebral palsy.
- dementia.
- epilepsy.
- motor neurone disease.
- multiple sclerosis (MS).
- Parkinson's Disease.
- spinal conditions.

Since 1990, the absolute number of individuals living with, or dying from, neurological conditions has increased. Parkinson's is the fastest-growing neurological condition in the world and currently, there is no cure. In Australia alone, 50 people are diagnosed with Parkinson's *every day*.

So why did I decide to write this book?

Being diagnosed with a neurological disorder is like being thrust into a foreign land without a map or translator. Suddenly, you're faced with an entirely new reality - one you never prepared for and certainly never wanted. The familiar landscape of your life is replaced by an intimidating terrain of medical jargon, treatment options and life-altering decisions.

In the aftermath of diagnosis, when your world feels like it's crumbling around you, you're expected to make choices that will profoundly impact your future. But how can you make informed decisions when you're still reeling from the news? When you're grappling with fear, anger and grief? It's a cruel irony that we're asked to be at our most rational and decisive during one of the most emotionally tumultuous periods of our lives.

In this vulnerable state, it's natural to cling to any sense of certainty or authority. Doctors become lifelines, their words carrying the weight of gospel. When you're staring your own mortality in the face, the promise of a treatment, any treatment, feels like a beacon of hope. You hang on every word, every recommendation, because what other choice do you have?

But should it be this way? Should we unquestioningly accept every word from our doctors as absolute truth?

Don't misunderstand me - medical professionals are invaluable allies in our health journey. Their expertise and dedication save lives every day. But they're human too, with their own biases, limitations and gaps in knowledge. While they're experts in medicine, we are the experts in our own bodies and lives.

I've come to believe that true health management requires a partnership between patient and doctor. It demands that we educate ourselves, ask questions, seek second opinions, explore all available options - conventional and alternative. It means acknowledging the emotional aspect of illness, not just the physical symptoms.

The path of a neurological disorder is challenging enough without the added burden of navigating it blindly. We need a medical system that empowers patients with knowledge, supports them emotionally and respects their autonomy. We need doctors who are *partners in our care*, not just providers of it.

Being diagnosed with a neurological disorder may thrust us into an unfamiliar world, but it doesn't mean we have to remain lost in it. By questioning, learning, advocating for ourselves, we can chart our own course through this new terrain. It's not an easy journey, but it's one where we can - and should - have a say in the direction we take.

I hope this book offers you a new point of view. When I was first diagnosed, I felt lost in a maze of medical jargon and overwhelming choices. I yearned for a guide that spoke to me not just as a patient, but as a person - someone grappling with fear, hope and everything in between. That's what I've aimed to create here.

I hope it educates you. Knowledge truly is power, especially when facing a neurological disorder. But I'm not just talking about memorizing symptoms or medication names. I mean real, practical knowledge. The kind that helps you understand your body, question your doctors (respectfully, of course), make informed decisions about your care. I've packed these pages with insights I wish I'd had from day one.

I hope this book inspires you. Living with a neurological disorder can sometimes feel like treading water in an endless ocean. But I promise you, there are islands of hope out there. I've shared stories of resilience, unexpected joys and small victories that felt as big as mountains. These aren't fairy tales of miracle cures, but real accounts of people living full, rich lives despite their diagnoses. Because that's possible for you too.

I hope it makes you laugh. Yes, laugh! Because if there's one thing I've learned, it's that humour can be the best medicine (well, after actual medicine, of course). I've included plenty of my own embarrassing moments and absurd situations that come with this territory. Because sometimes, when your body won't cooperate, laughter is the only sane response. Trust me, it feels good to laugh at the ridiculous dance we sometimes do with our own nervous systems.

But more importantly, I hope this book gives you choices. When I was diagnosed, I felt like my choices were being stripped away. But over time, I've discovered that there are always options - in treatment, in lifestyle, in outlook. I've laid out a buffet of possibilities here. Some might work for you, others might not and that's okay. The point is, you have the power to choose. You're not just a passive recipient of care, but an active participant in your own well-being.

This book isn't a replacement for medical advice and it certainly doesn't have all the answers. What it does have is a friend who's walked this path, stumbled, got back up and learned a thing or two along the way. It has permission to question, to explore, to hope. It has tools to help you navigate this new world you've been thrust into.

So dive in. Highlight, dog-ear, scribble in the margins. Use what serves you and discard what doesn't. This is your journey and while I can't walk it for you, I hope this book can be a companion along the way. Remember, you're not just living with a neurological disorder - you're living, period. There's still so much life to be lived.

Now, let's embark on this adventure together. Trust me, it's going to be one hell of a ride!

HOW IT ALL BEGAN

It all began on a quiet morning, I was savoring my breakfast, finding a moment of peace amidst the turmoil of a difficult marriage, when my left hand betrayed me with an unexpected tremor. I nearly spilled my coffee, but brushed it off as stress due to the complications in my life at that time. Oh, how we try to protect ourselves from the unknown.

As days turned to weeks and weeks to months, that small tremor ever so slowly grew into a constant companion. My dominant hand, once steady and sure, now struggled with life's simplest joys - stirring a cup of tea, applying mascara, buttoning a shirt. Every time I stepped outside, I felt a sense of dread. It wasn't the bustling streets or the crowded sidewalks that bothered me. It was my left hand—my rebellious, attention-seeking left hand.

It started subtly at first. A twitch here, a flick there. But soon, my hand developed a mind of its own. Whenever I walked down the street, it would start waving frantically, as if I was desperately trying to flag down every passerby.

The reactions varied. Some people smiled awkwardly and waved back, probably thinking I was just an overly friendly neighbor. Others looked confused, checking behind them to see if I was actually waving at someone else. The worst were those who frowned, clearly annoyed by my apparent need for attention.

I tried everything to control it. I'd shove my hand deep into my pocket, feeling the heat of embarrassment rise to my cheeks as I struggled to keep it contained. In restaurants, I'd sit on it, ignoring the strange looks from my dining companions as I shifted uncomfortably in my seat. During meetings, I'd keep it firmly planted under the table, gripping the edge so tightly my knuckles turned white.

My life became a constant battle against my own limb. I started to avoid going out altogether, dreading the moment when my hand would betray me again.

But as isolating as it was, I couldn't help but wonder—was my hand trying to tell me something? Was it reaching out for connections I was too afraid to make myself? Or was it simply a quirk of biology, a misfiring of neurons that had turned my everyday life into a comedy of errors?

Whatever the reason, one thing was clear: my left hand had become the director of my life's most awkward play and I was its unwilling star.
At home, away from prying eyes, I became my own mad scientist. My house transformed into a laboratory of adaptation, each room a new experiment in reclaiming control over my daily life.

I started in the kitchen. Weighted utensils became my new best friends. The extra heft helped steady my rebellious left hand, making meals less of a spectacle. Forks no longer launched food across the room and I could finally enjoy soup without wearing it.

In the bathroom, I embraced technology. An electric toothbrush buzzed away, doing most of the work while I focused on keeping my grip steady. Shaving became an adventure in ambidexterity, my right hand awkwardly learning the curves of my legs. Even the simplest acts of self-care had become herculean tasks. Washing my hair, once a mindless part of my routine, had transformed into a comedy of errors—or perhaps a tragedy, depending on my mood that day.

With my left hand waving and splashing uncontrollably, I'd end up with more shampoo on the walls and floor than in my hair. Rinsing was a game of chance, with water spraying everywhere except where I needed it. Don't even get me started on conditioning. More often than not, I'd emerge from the shower looking like I'd been caught in a particularly localised rainstorm.

Drying my hair was even worse. The hair dryer became a weapon of mass destruction in my hands—or rather, in my hand. I'd aim for my head, but my left hand would jerk, sending hot air blasting into my eyes or ears. On bad days, I'd give up and let my hair air dry, walking around with a damp head like I'd just emerged from a pool.

One frustrating morning, after a particularly disastrous attempt at hair care that left me looking like a half-drowned, lopsided poodle, I made a decision. Enough was enough.

I marched to the nearest hair salon, my left hand shoved deep in my pocket to avoid alarming the stylist. "Cut it off," I said, trying to sound more confident than I felt. "Short. Really short." The stylist raised an eyebrow but didn't question my sudden desire for a drastic change. As I watched my locks fall to the floor, I felt a mix of emotions—sadness at losing a part of my identity, but also a strange sense of liberation.

When it was done, I ran my right hand through my newly shorn hair. It was practical, easy to manage and required minimal styling. No more battles with the hairdryer, no more shampoo disasters .As I left the salon, I caught a glimpse of myself in a store window. The person staring back at me looked different—older, perhaps, or just changed. But there was a glint of determination in their eyes. This new hairstyle wasn't just about convenience; it was a symbol of my adaptability, my willingness to change in the face of adversity.

Dressing posed its own challenges. I hunted down shoes with velcro straps, bidding farewell to the daily struggle of lace-tying. Buttons became the enemy, I found myself gravitating towards pull-over shirts and elastic waistbands.

Almost without realizing it, I became adept at using my right hand for many tasks. It was a long, slow, hard process, but when faced with no choice, what else could I do? Some days, determination fueled me; others, I succumbed to tears of frustration. The simple act of writing my name became a monumental task, my signature transforming into an unrecognisable scrawl.

There were moments of triumph. The first time I successfully buttoned a shirt one-handed, I felt like I'd won an Olympic medal. But there were also days when the simplest tasks seemed insurmountable. I'd find myself staring at a jar of pickles, willing my left hand to cooperate, only to admit defeat and leave it unopened in the fridge.

Through it all, I learned patience. I discovered strengths I never knew I had. My right hand, once the silent partner in my daily activities, stepped up to the challenge. It learned to write, to cook, to tie shoelaces (on the rare occasions I dared to wear them).

Yet, even as I adapted, there was always that underlying current of frustration. Why me? Why my hand? But in the quiet moments, when I successfully completed a task that once seemed impossible, I felt a glimmer of pride. It wasn't the life I had imagined, but it was mine and I was learning to navigate it, one wobbly, waving step at a time.

As I look back now, I'm amazed at how I handled my emotions during those early years with Parkinson's. I recognize the strength it took, but at the time, I felt anything but strong. There were days when I felt utterly useless, questioning whether I wanted to continue living with this condition that was slowly reshaping my life. The future loomed before me, a terrifying unknown.

Thankfully, I wasn't alone in this battle. My family became my fortress, a strong team rallying around me. My husband, bless him, was an unwavering pillar of support. "Persevere, my darling," he'd say, his voice a soothing balm as I struggled with tasks that were once second nature. When I managed to complete them, his face would light up with pride, celebrating these small victories as if I'd conquered mountains.

I remember one evening, trying to put in earrings for a dinner out. My fingers trembled uncontrollably and the simple act of slipping the post through my earlobe became an insurmountable challenge. Frustration boiled over and I hurled the earrings across the room, collapsing onto the bed in tears. It was more than just about the jewelry; it was about losing the person I used to be. I was caught in limbo, mourning my old identity while not quite ready to accept the new one emerging from the tremors and tears.

My children, despite being in their late teens, struggled to reconcile the image of their strong, capable mother with this new reality. My daughter, in particular, found it difficult. She'd been used to seeing me as invincible and now she was faced with a mother who trembled constantly and often dissolved into tears. For quite a while, she stuck her head in the sand, unable or unwilling to learn about how Parkinson's would change my life—and by extension, hers. I couldn't blame her; I was barely coming to terms with it myself.

I tried to be strong for my family, to be the mother and wife they knew. But there were countless nights when the weight of it all became too much to bear. My husband would wake in the dark hours to find me lying on the floor, silently weeping for the life I was losing and the uncertain future ahead. He'd gather me in his arms, his presence a reminder that I wasn't facing this alone.

The journey towards acceptance was long (about two years) and fraught with setbacks. There were days when I felt I was making progress, only to be knocked back by a new symptom or limitation. But slowly, steadily, I began to find a level of acceptance. It wasn't resignation; rather, it was a hard-won peace with my new normal.

Looking back, I can see the strength it took to navigate those hard years. Each tremor, each tear, each moment of frustration was a step on the path to where I am now. I'm not the same person I was before Parkinson's entered my life, but I've discovered reserves of resilience I never knew I had.

My family has grown with me through this journey. My husband's unwavering support, my son's quiet understanding and my daughter's gradual acceptance have all been crucial parts of my story. Together, we've learned to adapt, to celebrate the good days and to face the challenges head-on.

This isn't the life I envisioned for myself, but it's mine. With each passing day, I'm learning to embrace it, tremors and all.

Away from my family's eyes, I scoured the internet, convincing myself it was just a vitamin deficiency or perhaps a pinched nerve. I increased my intake of B12, tried acupuncture and even resorted to old wives' tales involving apple cider vinegar.

The more I researched, the deeper I fell into a pit of anxiety. Every article I read seemed to point to worst-case scenarios and each podcast guest shared horror stories that left me trembling. I began to see symptoms everywhere – a slight headache became a potential brain tumor, a moment of forgetfulness morphed into early-onset dementia in my mind.

My days became consumed with symptom-checking and self-diagnosis. I'd wake up in the middle of the night, heart racing, convinced I'd discovered a new symptom or unexplained pain. I started keeping a journal of every physical sensation, no matter how minor, creating a chronicle of my spiraling fears.

Friends and family noticed the change in me. I'd cancel plans at the last minute, too anxious to leave the house or too busy following another lead on a medical forum. When I did socialise, I'd steer every conversation towards health topics, desperately seeking validation for my concerns or new information to add to my growing database of medical knowledge.

I knew, somewhere in the back of my mind, that this behavior wasn't healthy. But the fear of missing some crucial piece of information, some vital clue about my health, kept me locked in this cycle of endless searching and worrying. Anything to avoid facing the growing fear that something was seriously wrong.

As my symptoms grew and my wellness declined, I was counting the days to gain a solution. Each passing hour felt like an eternity, weighed down by the burden of uncertainty and fear. I marked off days on my calendar, not in anticipation of joyful events, but in a desperate countdown to my next doctor's appointment or test results.

My life became a series of waiting rooms and anxious phone calls. I'd stare at my phone, willing it to ring with news from the lab or the specialist's office. Every twinge or discomfort sent me spiraling into new theories and possibilities, each one more frightening than the last.

Sleep became elusive, replaced by long nights of tossing and turning, my mind racing through worst-case scenarios. When I did manage to drift off, my dreams were filled with hospitals and dire diagnoses. I'd wake up exhausted, both physically and emotionally, yet unable to escape the cycle of worry.

My relationships started to strain under the weight of my obsession. Friends grew distant, tired of my constant health talk and inability to engage in normal conversations. Family members walked on eggshells around me, never sure what might trigger a new bout of anxiety or send me rushing back to my computer for more frantic googling.

As the days ticked by, I felt myself slipping further away from the person I used to be. The search for a solution had become all-consuming, overshadowing every other aspect of my life. I longed for the day when I'd finally have answers, when I could breathe easily again and reclaim the parts of myself that had been lost in this maze of medical fears and endless research.

As I dutifully met with doctor after doctor, the world of medical terminology opened before me like a daunting maze. Brain lesions, Multiple Sclerosis, Parkinson's - such heavy words for such fragile hearts. The wait to see a neurologist felt endless, a year stretched thin by COVID's grasp. But hope has a way of surprising us.

That first neurologist's visit was a whirlwind of relief. As I walked down the corridor, tapped my fingers and counted backwards, I felt like I was passing a test I didn't know I was taking. "I have good news, not Parkinson's," she said, "just stress."

It was without a doubt my first experience of a lopsided attitude towards my medical journey. To have my illness almost shoved to the side with seemingly such simple tests worried me. The casual dismissal of my concerns by medical professionals left me feeling adrift and invalidated.

I had walked into the doctor's office armed with pages of notes, symptom logs and questions. But as the appointment progressed, I felt my voice growing smaller, my carefully prepared points dissolving under the brisk efficiency of the consultation. The doctor's apparent lack of concern felt like a slap in the face after months of my own intense worry and research.

As I left the clinic, prescription in hand for tests that seemed far too basic given the complexity of my symptoms, a new kind of fear set in. What if they were missing something crucial? What if these "simple" tests weren't enough to uncover the real problem?

The disconnect between my lived experience and the medical response was jarring. I felt caught between two worlds - the intense, all-consuming reality of my symptoms and fears and the seemingly nonchalant approach of the healthcare system. This disparity only fueled my anxiety further, convincing me that I needed to push harder, research more and become my own advocate in a system that didn't seem to fully hear me.

That night, as I stared at the ceiling, unable to sleep, I realised that this journey was going to be more complicated than I had initially thought. It wasn't just about finding a diagnosis or cure anymore; it was about navigating a complex medical landscape while holding onto my own truth and experiences. It was my first step towards truly listening to my body and advocating for myself.

Seeking a second opinion was an act of self-love, though I didn't realise it at the time. The next neurologist was quick with his diagnosis and quicker with his prescription pad. His cold manner and lack of empathy were a stark reminder of how vulnerable we can feel in the face of illness. I will never forget how dazed I was during that appointment. I took the medication obediently, wanting so desperately to trust in the system designed to heal us.

It wasn't until the medication began to fight against me that I found my true strength.The side effects of the medication became far less tolerable than my illness. As I researched my condition further, each piece of information became a stepping stone on a path to understanding. This journey, born from necessity, blossomed into something beautiful - a chance to reclaim my health, to listen to my body and to become my own advocate.

Now, as I write these words, I'm filled with a profound sense of purpose. This book isn't just my story; it's a love letter to everyone facing their own health battles. It's a reminder that within each of us lies the power to question, to learn and to heal. My trembling hand led me to a trembling soul, but together, we found strength. In sharing this journey, I hope to hold space for others to find their strength too.

MY INITIAL PARKINSON'S DIAGNOSIS

In the sterile confines of a cold examination room, my entire world shattered with the precision of a surgeon's scalpel. "You have Parkinson's," the doctor's words felt like a crushing blow, each syllable a nail in the coffin of my former life. At only 48 years old, I suddenly found myself standing on the precipice of an abyss I never knew existed. What did this devastating diagnosis mean for me and my future? The depth of devastation and shock that comes with a life-altering diagnosis like Parkinson's is truly impossible to capture in words. The very foundations of our lives, our sense of security and certainty, can be shattered in an instant.

We go through life, often taking our health and our futures for granted, focused on making the most of each day. Then, in a cruel twist of fate, that carefully crafted reality is snatched away, leaving us stranded in a strange new world we never could have imagined. The overwhelming emotions - the grief, the fear, the sense of loss - can be truly crippling in that moment.

No matter how eloquently one tries to describe it, the true experience of that earth-shattering diagnosis can only be understood by those who have lived it. The abrupt transition from carefree normalcy to uncertain new normal is a visceral, all-consuming experience that defies simple explanation. It's a rupture in the fabric of one's life that leaves an indelible mark, changing a person irrevocably.

No words can truly do justice to the sheer devastation of that pivotal moment. It's a shattering of assumptions, a loss of innocence that leaves the individual grappling with a new and terrifying reality. The trauma of that diagnosis lingers, manifesting in ways both obvious and subtle, as the person struggles to redefine their identity and reimagine their future. It's a profound experience.

"We'll try to get you to 70," the doctor continued, his tone as casual and indifferent as if he were discussing the weather. "Take this medication. Make another appointment in 3 months." Then, with a callousness that bordered on cruelty, I waited with bated breath for him to utter the final blow, perhaps saying "I'm off to play golf now."

In that agonizing moment, time seemed to freeze. The air grew thick, suffocating me with the crushing weight of an uncertain future. Shock? No, that word was far too mild to capture the seismic shift that had just occurred. My mind reeled, desperately grasping for understanding amidst the whirlwind of medical jargon and life-altering implications.

The relisation crashed over me like a tidal wave, each sob wracking my body with the force of shattered dreams. My husband, my rock through so many storms, now seemed distant on the shore of a future I could no longer clearly see. How would this change us? Would he still see me as the woman he fell in love with, or would I become a burden, a patient instead of a partner? The uncertainty haunts me to this day.

Oh, my precious children. Their faces flashed before my eyes, a montage of first steps, school plays and tender hugs. I had always imagined being there for every milestone, cheering them on as they navigated life's twists and turns. Now, doubt and uncertainty clouded those cherished visions. Would I be able to dance at their weddings? To offer the advice and comfort they would need most?

But it was the dream of being a grandmother that truly broke my heart. I had held onto that vision for so long - of chasing little ones through the park, baking cookies together, reading bedtime stories with silly voices. It was meant to be a time of joy, of second chances to savor all the small moments that slip by so quickly when you're a busy parent. The thought that I might not be able to be that active, doting grandmother I had always imagined felt like losing a piece of my future self.

As the tears flowed, I felt the full depth of my grief. It wasn't just about the physical changes or the medical diagnosis. It was mourning for a life I had planned, for a future that now seemed hazy and uncertain. They say with Parkinson's that it is a continuous grieving process and I wholeheartedly agree. Each day when your body lets you down by not being able to do another simple task is another day of profound sorrow.

In that moment of raw vulnerability, I made a silent promise to myself and to my loved ones. Whatever challenges lay ahead, I would face them with all the love and courage I could muster. The journey might look different than I had imagined, but the destination - a life filled with love and meaningful connections - remained the same.

Whether it's Parkinson's creeping through my nervous system, cancer ravaging cells with reckless abandon, or some obscure malady lurking in the shadows of medical textbooks, a life-changing diagnosis is a brutal awakening. It's a moment that separates your life into "before" and "after," leaving you stranded in a no man's land of fear and uncertainty.

I look back now and vividly remember the doctor's words - "Parkinson's is very subjective", "It's hard to diagnose", "The shade of gray in your MRI can be read different ways by different people." Even as he expressed that level of uncertainty, I still sat there as if he were the god of medicine, someone whose every word I was to accept without question.

I am still utterly astounded at myself for the way I blindly accepted that medication prescription the doctor handed me that day. I didn't question anything - not a single word he said, not the ambiguity he'd expressed about the Parkinson's diagnosis, not the implications of what starting that treatment regime would mean for my life going forward. I simply resigned myself to the fact that I was now firmly in the hands of the medical profession, relinquishing my own agency and autonomy without a second thought.

It's an unsettling relisation, to recognize how easily I handed over that control, that autonomy, in the face of a life-altering diagnosis. I allowed myself to be completely subsumed by the perceived authority of the doctor, even as he himself acknowledged the subjectivity and ambiguity underlying his pronouncement. I was so desperate to cling to some semblance of certainty that I forsook my own instincts and decision-making power.I abdicated my own intuition and simply accepted the verdict, even as a sliver of doubt lingered. The perceived power and infallibility of the white-coated professional overwhelmed any inclination I might have had to assert my own voice, to demand more clarity or explore alternative perspectives.

Now, looking back on that pivotal experience, I recognize the complex power dynamics at play in the doctor-patient relationship. I see how we are so often conditioned to comply and defer, even when the certainty being conveyed is tinged with ambiguity. That day, I willingly placed my life in the hands of someone who openly acknowledged the subjectivity and uncertainty inherent in the diagnosis - and yet, I still accepted it without question.

This relisation has been a profound one for me. It has highlighted the urgent need for a fundamental shift in how we approach healthcare, one that truly empowers patients to be active participants in their own care. We must find the courage to question, to challenge and to assert our right to a medical experience that aligns with our values and needs, even in our most vulnerable moments.

What I began to realise over time is that my mind and my body are my own. I control the outcome of this journey far more than any doctor ever could. As knowledgeable and skilled as these medical professionals may be, they can never fully see, feel or touch the sheer determination that I can summon up from the depths of my being.

It was a shift in perspective for me - recognising that the true locus of control lies within me, not in the hands of those white-coated authorities. No matter how dire the diagnosis, no matter how bleak the prognosis, I possess an innate power and agency that transcends the limitations they might try to impose.

Far too often, patients like myself are conditioned to view doctors as the sole arbiters of our health and wellbeing, relinquishing our own authority in the process. But I've learned that this mindset is a disservice to our inherent capacity for resilience, adaptation and self-directed healing. Our minds and our bodies are our own - we are not beholden to the constraints of a medical label or treatment plan.

This awareness has been truly transformative for me. It has empowered me to approach my healthcare journey as an active participant, rather than a passive recipient of care. I no longer resign myself to the limitations that others try to place upon me. Instead, I draw upon an unshakable well of determination, fueled by the knowledge that I hold the power to shape my own path forward.

Of course, the medical professionals still play a vital role - their expertise and guidance are invaluable. But I've come to see them as partners in my healing, not the sole decision-makers. I engage with them as an equal, questioning, challenging and collaborating to find solutions that truly resonate with my needs and values.

This shift in perspective has been nothing short of liberating. It has allowed me to approach each obstacle, each new symptom or setback, with a fierce resolve. I am no longer defined by my diagnosis, but rather empowered by the conviction that I can overcome, adapt and redefine what's possible, regardless of the challenges that may arise.

As I left the doctor's office that day, the world outside seemed alien. People walked by, laughing, living, oblivious to the fact that my universe had just imploded. I was now an unwilling member of a club no one wanted to join, facing a future I never imagined, armed with nothing but a prescription and the echoing words of a doctor more concerned with his tee time than the life he had just upended.

The stark reality is indeed harrowing and, sadly, all too common. The blind faith we place in medical professionals, born of desperation and societal conditioning, leads us down a path of unquestioning compliance. Test after test, each one a nail in the coffin of our former life, each visit to the doctor a grim reminder of our new reality. The sterile walls of the examination room became the boundaries of my new world, closing in with each visit.

The medications, promised as salvation, became a cruel joke. Side effects worse than the original symptoms plagued me, chaining me to a regime that seemed to offer more suffering than relief. I've suffered through ulcers in my mouth, debilitating dryness that made swallowing a painful ordeal, agonizing cuts on my lips - the list goes on. These were not just minor annoyances, but truly debilitating symptoms that robbed me of my ability to even perform the most basic functions, like eating and sleeping. Pills became both my lifeline and my prison, marking the hours of my days with bitter reminders of my condition.

Through it all, the doctor - that figure that I was taught to revere and trust - offered no solace. No warm hand of comfort, no words of encouragement. Just cold, clinical phrases. My journey - from the shock of diagnosis, through the maze of tests and treatments, to the grim relisation of a life forever changed - is a poignant testament to the often-overlooked human cost of illness. It's a stark reminder of the gap between medical treatment and true healing, between managing a condition and nurturing a person.

My experience raises questions about our healthcare system, the doctor-patient relationship and how we as a society deal with chronic illness and disability. It's a call for more compassion, more holistic care and a reminder that behind every diagnosis is a human being and their loved ones grappling with an entirely new reality.

"Do you choose to accept this diagnosis?" - it's a question that defies the traditional doctor-patient dynamic. It implies that even in the face of a devastating medical verdict, we retain agency. It's a battle cry against resignation, a refusal to be defined solely by a medical label. It suggests a radical shift in perspective - one that places power back into the hands of the patient.

This phrase opens up a world of possibilities:

1. It questions the infallibility of medical diagnoses.
2. It empowers patients to seek second opinions, explore alternative treatments, or delve into cutting-edge research.
3. It challenges the notion that a diagnosis is a sentence, suggesting instead that it's a starting point for a new journey which offers us far more value. Years later, I can attest this to be true.
4. It encourages a proactive approach to health, where the patient becomes an active participant in their care rather than a passive recipient.

The implications of this mindset are profound. It could mean:

- Seeking out multiple medical opinions. I strongly agree with this and saw numerous doctors until I found one that demonstrated that he was keen to work *with* me and not talk at me.
- Exploring both conventional and alternative therapies. I have become an advocate for this and indeed this is what this book is all about.
- Diving deep into the latest research on your condition. We are blessed that we have so much information at our fingertips.
- Connecting with others who have defied similar diagnoses. Once again, we are fortunate that many social media channels allow us to become part of a community.
- Focusing on overall well-being rather than just managing symptoms. Looking back on my journey, I am now much more aware and proactive in all areas of my health - I just wish I had had this focus prior to my Parkinson's diagnosis!

This approach doesn't deny the reality of the condition, but it refuses to let that condition define one's entire existence. It's about reclaiming control in a situation where you might feel powerless.

I remember early on in my diagnosis, listening to a podcast and someone said "Parkinson's gives you more than it takes away from you". At the time, I thought it was a cruel joke, however when I look at my wellness, my community and understanding of life now, I believe that statement to be true!

"Do you choose to accept this diagnosis?" - it's an invitation to fight, to hope, to redefine what's possible. It's a reminder that even in our darkest moments, we have choices. Sometimes, choosing not to accept the limitations others place on us can be the first step towards a different kind of healing.

Do we surrender to the comforting embrace of conventional wisdom, or do we dare to blaze our own trail through the wilderness of alternative therapies? The clock ticks, the pressure mounts and the world holds its breath, waiting for our decision.

IS MEDICATION THE ONLY ANSWER?

In this moment of crisis, we are forced to confront the terrifying truth: our health, our very lives, hang in the balance. The choice we make here, in the shadow of diagnosis, will echo through every remaining day of our existence. In the wake of that earth-shattering diagnosis, as the dust of shattered dreams begins to settle, we find ourselves standing at a crossroads. The path before us, once clear and certain, now splinters into a labyrinth of choices, each fraught with consequence.

On one side looms the towering edifice of Western medicine, its sterile halls echoing with the promise of scientific certainty. We've been conditioned since birth to view doctors as infallible deities in white coats, their words gospel, their prescriptions our salvation. It's the safe choice, the expected choice - to bow our heads and swallow the bitter pills of conformity.

But as we stand on this precipice, a chilling relisation dawns. Can these doctors, these strangers in sterile rooms, truly know the intricate landscape of our minds and bodies? Can a few hurried minutes and a battery of tests capture the essence of our being? Does it really matter?

Then there's the Faustian bargain of medication - a devil's contract written in fine print. Relief comes at a cost, each pill a double-edged sword. The very treatment meant to save us might become our undoing, its side effects a cascade of new torments, sometimes eclipsing the very ailment they were meant to cure. This, like many, I experienced first hand!

Every time I tried to advocate for myself, to voice my concerns and questions about this diagnosis, the medical establishment responded with the same dismissive refrain: "There is no cure", "Just focus on quality of life" and the automatic prescription of medication without any real understanding of what my life was actually like.

It was deeply frustrating and disheartening to feel so completely disregarded and misunderstood. Instead of engaging with me as a whole person, with unique needs and perspectives, the doctors seemed to view me solely through the lens of my Parkinson's diagnosis. Every inquiry, every attempt to better comprehend the implications of this condition, was met with another pill to swallow, another pharmaceutical "solution" that failed to address the core of my struggles.

The implication that depression was an inevitability, without any exploration of alternative approaches or coping strategies, was a glaring oversight that speaks to the systemic failures within our healthcare system. I deserved so much more than to have my concerns dismissed and my agency undermined by an over-reliance on medication. Even years after my Parkinson's diagnosis, I still find myself running into the same old problem when talking to certain doctors about the progression of my disease - the dreaded "double your medication" response.

It's as if they have a one-size-fits-all prescription pad and the only solution they can muster is to simply increase the dosage of my Parkinson's drugs. Never mind the potential side effects, the impact on my carefully crafted holistic routine, or the fact that I've already tried that approach to diminishing returns.

This experience leaves me feeling profoundly disillusioned with the medical establishment's approach to chronic illness. Rather than empowering me as an active partner in my own care, they seemed content to reduce my experience to a checklist of symptoms to be managed through a one-size-fits-all regime. There was no genuine attempt to understand the nuances of my situation, the specific ways in which Parkinson's was impacting my daily life and overall well-being.

However, the decision to step off the well-worn path of conventional medicine as the overall answer is not one made lightly. It's a choice that requires courage, a willingness to question the status quo and often, a leap of faith into the unknown. As I contemplated this journey, I felt the weight of responsibility not just for my own health, but for the hopes and fears of those who love me.

I thought of my husband, his worry lines deepening with each new symptom, each failed treatment. Of my children, their young faces etched with a concern no child should have to bear for a parent. They too were on this journey with me, their lives irrevocably altered by my condition. Their support was unwavering, but I could see the toll it took on them - the sleepless nights, the researching of symptoms, the silent prayers for a miracle cure.

Did I have the right to blindly follow the medical authorities and simply comply with their prescribed medication regime? Or did I have the agency to risk a more holistic approach, even in the face of such a daunting diagnosis? These were the questions that weighed heavily on my mind as I grappled with the implications of my Parkinson's diagnosis.

Ultimately, swallowing a pill – it's a momentary act, a fleeting second where we can pretend we've taken control. The tiny capsule slides down our throat and with it, we gulp down the illusion of proactivity. The ease of medication is a siren's song, lulling us into complacency. No sweat, no strain, no soul-searching required. Just open, swallow, repeat. It's a passive surrender disguised as treatment, a capitulation masked as care.

What of the treatments? Those sterile rooms where we lay our bodies down, offering ourselves up like sacrifices on the altar of modern medicine. We arrive, docile and compliant, ready to be poked, prodded and processed. Our agency checked at the door, we become mere vessels for procedures, our voices silenced in the face of medical authority.

This effortless acquiescence demands nothing of our spirit, asks nothing of our will. We don't have to dig deep, don't have to question and don't have to face the terrifying possibility that healing might require more than what comes in a bottle or through an IV.

The hard truth is that real healing – deep, transformative healing – is often a grueling journey. It demands we look inward, confront our demons, overhaul our lifestyles. It asks us to question everything we thought we knew about health, about our bodies, about ourselves.

But that path is steep, fraught with uncertainty. It requires a strength many of us fear we don't possess. So instead, we opt for the easy way out. We choose the pill, the treatment, the abdication of responsibility. In doing so, we may be choosing to remain prisoners of our diagnosis, forever bound to a system that treats us not as individuals with unique stories and struggles, but as walking manifestations of a medical textbook.

Could the answer be as simple as doctors becoming more curious?

"Hello Lisa, it's so good to check in with you today. How are you feeling? I want you to know that I'm here to listen, without any judgment and to learn more about your personal journey."

"What's most important to you as you navigate this path with Parkinson's? I imagine there are many aspects - physical, emotional, spiritual - that you're trying to balance. Tell me more about what matters most to you right now."

"And your care team - can you share a bit about who makes up that support network for you? Do you feel they've taken the time to truly understand you as a whole person, beyond just the medical diagnosis? I'm curious to hear your perspective on how they approach your care."

"How is your partner and family doing? Do you feel that they need additional support?"

"Exercise and diet are so crucial for managing Parkinson's symptoms. What does your personal routine look like? Are you able to stay active in ways that feel nourishing for both your body and mind? How about your diet - have you explored any specific nutritional approaches that have been helpful?"

"I also want to ask about alcohol consumption. I know that can be a sensitive topic, but I'm genuinely interested in understanding your relationship with it, if you're comfortable sharing. Does it play a role, positive or negative, in your daily life?"

"The most important thing is for me to learn about you as an individual - your values, your goals, your unique circumstances. I want to understand the full picture, not just the medical details. Please feel free to share as much or as little as you'd like. I'm here to listen, support and walk alongside you on this journey."..... Said no doctor ever.

Curious questions are almost never asked!

IS THERE ANOTHER WAY?

Indeed, there's no shame in embracing only Western medicine if it aligns with your beliefs and needs. For many, it offers a path to improved quality of life and management of health conditions. The decision to take medication is deeply personal and shouldn't be subject to outside judgment.

The mind-body connection is powerful, and sometimes the very act of taking medication – combined with the belief in its efficacy – can contribute to positive outcomes. This doesn't diminish the real physiological effects of medications, but highlights the complex interplay between our beliefs and our physical responses.

1. Challenge your doctor

Actively engaging with and challenging your doctor is a crucial part of being an empowered patient. This doesn't mean being confrontational, but rather approaching the relationship as a collaborative partnership. Some key ways to challenge your doctor include:

- Asking questions to fully understand your condition, treatment options and rationale for recommendations
- Expressing concerns about proposed treatments, such as side effects or how they may impact your holistic wellness approach
- Advocating for alternative or complementary therapies that align with your personal preferences and needs
- Requesting a second opinion if you're unsure about a diagnosis or treatment plan
- Pushing back politely but firmly if a doctor seems unwilling to consider your perspective and experiences

The goal is to ensure your healthcare decisions are well-informed and tailored to your unique circumstances, rather than simply deferring to the doctor's authority. I am at the point where I produce a plan to my doctors that I have researched and know will work for me and my lifestyle and basically just get their sign off after a mutually respectful discussion!

2. **Question facts**

While respecting the medical expertise of your healthcare providers, it's valuable to maintain a critical mindset and seek deeper understanding. This involves:

- Researching your condition and treatment options from reputable sources, so much easier to do with the internet and support groups on socials.
- Asking clarifying questions when medical information is presented
- Discussing your findings and perspectives with your doctor
- Being open to challenging conventional wisdom if your personal experience suggests alternative approaches may be more effective

Questioning facts doesn't mean rejecting medical advice, but rather striving to be an active, informed partner in your care. This can lead to more nuanced and personalised treatment plans.

3. **Own your health Journey**

Taking responsibility for your physical, mental, and emotional well-being is empowering and can significantly improve healthcare outcomes. This includes:

- Practicing self-care through lifestyle modifications like diet, exercise and stress management
- closely monitoring your symptoms and maintaining detailed records

- Researching and implementing complementary therapies that align with your values
- Communicating openly with your healthcare team about your needs and preferences
- Making informed decisions about treatments, rather than passively deferring
- Advocating for yourself when faced with dismissive or insensitive responses from providers

Owning your health journey demonstrates your commitment to wellness and positions you as an equal partner in the process.

4. Share experiences

Open and honest communication with your healthcare providers about your lived experiences is essential for developing effective, personalised treatment plans. This includes:

- Discussing the nuances of your symptoms, including how they fluctuate and impact your daily life
- Sharing the emotional and psychological tolls of your condition
- Describing the benefits and drawbacks you've experienced with various treatments
- Expressing your goals, fears and priorities regarding your health and quality of life
- Providing feedback on how well interventions are working (or not working) for you

By sharing these intimate details, you can help your healthcare team gain a more holistic understanding of your situation and tailor their recommendations accordingly.

5. **Guide your care**

While your doctors have valuable medical expertise, you are the expert on your own body and lived experiences. Approaching the relationship as a partnership can lead to better outcomes:

- Collaborating with your healthcare team to set treatment goals and priorities
- Providing input on the feasibility and acceptability of proposed interventions
- Suggesting adjustments to the care plan based on your unique needs and preferences
- Taking an active role in decision-making, rather than just deferring to your provider's recommendations
- Maintaining open communication about the successes and challenges of your treatment journey
- Providing constructive feedback to improve the quality of your care

This guiding role acknowledges the vital contribution of your personal expertise and ensures your healthcare aligns with your holistic wellness goals.

There are two crucial aspects that we must keep front of mind:

1. **Don't Feel Guilty for Using Your Allotted Time**

It's important to remember that you have a right to the full attention of your healthcare providers, even if that means your appointment extends beyond the typical 15-20 minute slot. You may wait months to see your neurologist, so it's crucial that you make the most of that limited facetime.

Far too often, patients feel pressured to rush through their concerns or cut themselves short in order to keep the appointment "on schedule." But the reality is, your health and wellbeing should be the top priority, not arbitrary time constraints.

When you have a complex, chronic condition like Parkinson's, there are inevitably going to be nuances, fluctuations, and multifaceted concerns that require more in-depth discussion. Forcing yourself to squeeze everything into a brief window does a disservice to your care.

Instead, be upfront with your neurologist about needing a bit more time. Acknowledge the busy schedule, but assert your need to fully address your current status and needs. Most providers will understand and accommodate, as long as you're respectful of their other commitments.

Remember, you are not just a patient - you are a partner in your own healthcare. As a partner, you deserve to have your voice heard and your experiences validated, even if that means the appointment runs a few minutes long. Don't feel guilty about taking the time you require.

2. Maintain an Open Mind

Never go into a medical appointment with a closed mind. While it's understandable to be skeptical of treatments or approaches that seem unfamiliar or unorthodox, rigidly dismissing them can prevent you from discovering potentially life-changing solutions.

Sometimes the most transformative answers lie outside the realm of conventional medicine. Keeping an open mind allows you to consider a wider array of therapies, from complementary treatments to lifestyle modifications, that may profoundly enhance your overall wellbeing.

This doesn't mean blindly accepting every suggestion your providers make. It's still important to question, research and advocate for what feels right for you. But approaching appointments with curiosity and a willingness to learn can open the door to unexpected breakthroughs.

Perhaps your neurologist mentions a new exercise program you've never tried. Or your physical therapist proposes integrating mindfulness techniques into your routine. By entering the conversation without preconceptions, you create space for innovative, personalised approaches that may be exactly what your mind and body need.

Cultivating this open mindset requires ongoing practice and self-awareness. It means acknowledging your own biases and actively working to expand your perspective. But the payoff can be tremendous, leading to more collaborative, fulfilling partnerships with your healthcare team.

Remember, your Parkinson's journey is uniquely yours. By honouring the time you need and keeping an open mind, you empower yourself to find the most comprehensive, effective solutions - ones that may just surprise and delight you.

By embracing these approaches - challenging your doctor, questioning facts, owning your health, sharing experiences and guiding your care - you can become a true partner in managing your journey. This empowered mindset, combined with your medical team's expertise, can lead to more effective, personalised and satisfying healthcare outcomes.

This strikes a balance between respecting medical science and empowering individuals to be active participants in their healthcare decisions. It's a call for informed choice and personalised medicine, recognising that health is not just about treating symptoms, but about aligning care with an individual's overall life goals and values.

HOW I ACCIDENTLY FOUND ALTERNATIVE THERAPIES

My journey seems to reflect a profound and increasingly common experience in healthcare. It's a testament to the growing recognition that health is far more complex than a series of symptoms to be treated with medication.

Fortunately for me, a friend of mine invited me to a Parkinson's retreat and the day I arrived, I had no idea my life was about to change forever. Looking back, I can still feel the mixture of skepticism and nervousness churning in my stomach as I arrived. I was a facts-and-figures person, clinging to the safety of medical journals and prescription bottles. The idea of "holistic wellness" seemed like New Age nonsense to me then – how naive I was!

As I pulled up to the retreat centre, my heart sank. This was no posh hotel; it was more like a rustic summer camp for adults. I felt like Maria in "The Sound of Music," but not the joyful, singing-on-the-hillside Maria. No, I was Maria staring wide-eyed at the convent gates, wondering what on earth I'd gotten myself into. The spartan single beds, shared kitchen and distinct lack of modern amenities made me want to turn tail and run.

But I stayed. Oh, am I grateful I did.

Those four days cracked open my heart in ways I never expected. As I fumbled through my first meditation session, I felt a strange sense of peace wash over me – a feeling I hadn't experienced since my diagnosis. The gentle movements of yoga brought tears to my eyes as I reconnected with a body I'd started to view as my enemy.

But it was the connections with my fellow "parkies" that truly shattered my defenses. Sitting around the dinner table, sharing vegan meals and our deepest fears, I finally felt seen. These people understood the terror of a hand that wouldn't stop shaking, the frustration of a mind that sometimes betrayed you. We laughed, we cried and we formed bonds that would become my lifeline in the years to come.

Each new experience – from mindfulness walks in the woods to late-night conversations under the stars – chipped away at the walls I'd built around myself. I found myself opening up, not just to new ideas, but to a new way of seeing the world and my place in it.

I never thought I'd find myself lying on a table, surrounded by the gentle chimes of exotic instruments and the soothing scent of essential oils. Yet there I was, eyes covered, surrendering myself to a practice I knew little about - sound healing. It was a leap of faith, born from a newfound openness to alternative approaches in my journey with Parkinson's.

As the healer worked his magic, I felt an unusual combination of deep relaxation and acute awareness. The pain in my tremoring arm intensified to an almost unbearable level and I was on the verge of calling it quits. But something held me back - an instinct that this pain was necessary, that it was leading to something important.

Then it happened. As the healer's hands rested on my head, I felt a primal roar building from the depths of my being. It wasn't just a sound - it was a physical sensation, as if years of pent-up pain and frustration were finally finding release. Like a bear emerging from hibernation, this roar seemed to embody every struggle, every setback, every moment of anguish I'd ever experienced.

The release felt endless, but also incredibly soothing. It was as if each second of that roar was washing away layers of emotional debris, leaving me lighter and clearer. When it was over, I felt transformed. It's hard to explain, but I truly believe that in that moment, my soul was cleansed, making room for a new strength and determination to face Parkinson's head-on.

This experience changed me profoundly. I walked away feeling unburdened, with a renewed sense of purpose and hope. It opened my eyes to the power of alternative healing methods and the importance of addressing not just the physical, but also the emotional and spiritual aspects of living with a chronic condition.

While I still rely on my conventional treatments, this experience has become a cornerstone in my approach to managing Parkinson's. It reminds me daily that healing can come in unexpected forms and that sometimes, the most powerful medicine is allowing ourselves to feel, release and transform.

By the time I left, I felt raw and vulnerable, but also strangely whole. It was as if I'd shed a skin I no longer needed. The skeptic in me was still there, but she'd been joined by a part of me that recognised the power of connection, of stillness, of treating my body and soul with kindness.

Now, years later, I still get a lump in my throat when I think about that first retreat. I've returned many times since, each visit feeling like coming home. The simple rooms that once seemed so stark now feel like a warm embrace. The lack of TV and cell service, once so daunting, now feels like blessed relief from the noise of the world.

Most profound of all is the shift in how I see my place in the universe. Where I once felt isolated in my diagnosis, I now feel deeply connected – to nature, to my fellow human beings, to the rhythm of life itself. There's a bittersweet beauty in this journey. Parkinson's has taken things from me, yes, but it's also given me a depth of experience and emotion I never knew was possible.

Every time I practice meditation or prepare a nourishing plant-based meal, I feel a surge of gratitude for that scared, skeptical woman who took a chance on a retreat all those years ago. She had no idea she was taking the first steps towards not just managing her condition, but towards a richer, more meaningful life.

So as I explored various wellness approaches, I've come to realise that the combination of traditional and non-traditional methods works best for me. In today's society, we're seeing an increasing trend towards holistic treatments, with many people opting exclusively for alternative therapies. However, my personal journey has led me to appreciate the value of a balanced approach.

This journey hasn't always been easy. There are still days when I rage against my diagnosis, when the future feels terrifying. But now I have tools to weather those storms. More than that, I have a community that holds me up when I falter and a deep well of inner strength I never knew I possessed.

My Parkinson's journey has become a spiritual awakening, a path to self-discovery that I never could have imagined. It's taught me that true healing goes far beyond pills and doctor's visits. It's about finding harmony – with our bodies, with nature, with each other. In that harmony, I've found a peace and purpose that no diagnosis can shake.

Through my research and personal experiences, I've found that integrating conventional medicine with complementary therapies offers me the most comprehensive care. This balanced strategy allows me to benefit from the rigorous scientific approach of traditional medicine while also embracing the holistic perspective of alternative treatments.

For instance, I might use conventional medicine for diagnosis and treatment of specific conditions (like stiffness and rigidity), while incorporating practices like acupuncture, meditation, or herbal remedies to support my overall well-being and manage stress. This integrated approach has helped me address both the symptoms and root causes of health issues, leading to better overall outcomes.

I believe that this balanced method allows me to take advantage of the strengths of both worlds. While I respect those who choose to go down the path of holistic treatment only, I've found that for me, the synergy between traditional and non-traditional approaches provides the most effective and satisfying wellness plan.

My experience highlights several crucial points:

1. Holistic approach

I recognised that wellness extends beyond "popping pills," encompassing a broader understanding of health that includes physical, mental and possibly spiritual aspects.

2. Limitations of traditional medical encounters

Short appointments often fail to capture the full complexity of a patient's life and experiences, especially with chronic or progressive conditions like Parkinson's.

3. Personal expertise

Living with a progressive disability gave me insights that even well-trained doctors couldn't fully grasp without my input. Not to mention all symptoms are different for all.

4. Existential questioning

Facing significant health challenges often leads to deeper introspection about life's meaning and purpose, regardless of one's spiritual inclinations.

5. Self-advocacy and research

I took the initiative to educate myself, empowering me to engage more actively in my healthcare decisions.

6. Challenging the status quo

By presenting alternative options to my doctors, I was participating in a broader shift towards more collaborative, patient-centered care. I support this whole heartedly.

My approach - combines respect for medical expertise with proactive self-education and advocacy - represents a powerful model for patient engagement. It acknowledges the value of medical science while also recognising its limitations, especially in addressing the unique, lived experiences of individuals with chronic conditions.

This kind of informed, assertive patient involvement can lead to more personalised and effective treatment plans. It also challenges healthcare providers to stay current with emerging therapies, to truly listen to their patients' experiences and insights.

My journey is a compelling reminder that patients are not just passive recipients of care, but active partners in their own health journeys. It's an approach that can lead to more satisfying and potentially more effective healthcare experiences, especially for those dealing with complex, long-term health challenges.

By combining these four elements with traditional medical approaches, I crafted a personalised wellness strategy that addresses the complexity of human health. I do not suggest this for everyone, I am simply detailing where I and my family focused our energy.

Let's delve into this transformative quartet with more to come later:

1. Meditation

The silent warrior in my arsenal. Through the stillness of mind, I found a sanctuary amidst the chaos of symptoms and treatments. Meditation doesn't just calm the mind; it rewires it, potentially altering pain perception and boosting emotional resilience. I came to learn that meditating allows the body to rest and repair. The most exciting thing for me is when I meditate, my symptoms stop. I get a break from my tremor in my hand, my leg doesn't shake and the pain in my muscles goes away. Even for the briefest of time, it is more than worth it!

2. Neuroplasticity

Here's where I became the architect of my own brain. By harnessing the brain's ability to form new neural connections, I was rewiring pathways affected by my condition. It's a rebellion against the notion of fixed limitations, a declaration that change is possible at the most fundamental level. I became so fascinated with the brain's ability to rewire itself that I am now a Certified Mind-Body Practitioner. Firing and connecting new neurons in my brain is front of mind everyday all day for me, I honestly believe that I can rewire my brain to remove Parkinson's.

3. **Diet**

Food becomes medicine. Every meal is a choice, a chance to nourish or neglect. By taking control of my nutrition, I was not just feeding my body; I was potentially influencing inflammation, energy levels and even the course of my condition. I delve further into this as there is much discussion around diet, especially vegan vs carnivore!

4. **Exercise**

Movement as defiance against limitations. Each step, stretch, or lift is a testament to your body's enduring strength. Exercise isn't just about physical fitness; it's a potent mood enhancer, stress reliever and possible symptom mitigator. If we don't keep on using our body, we will lose the ability to do so.

By interweaving these elements with my medical treatments, I created a tapestry of care that addresses body, mind and spirit. This approach acknowledges the complex interplay between physical symptoms, mental state and overall well-being.

My strategy embodies the essence of integrative medicine, combining the best of conventional treatments with evidence-based complementary therapies. It's a bold statement that healing is not a passive process, but an active engagement with all aspects of one's health.

This multifaceted approach doesn't just treat symptoms; it cultivates resilience, fosters a sense of contro, and potentially improves overall quality of life. It's a testament to the power of taking charge of one's health journey, of becoming not just a patient, but a partner in the healing process.

My experience serves as a reminder that even in the face of progressive conditions, there are always avenues to explore, always ways to influence our well-being. It's a call to others to look beyond the prescription pad, to embrace a more comprehensive view of health and healing.

MEDITATION

Meditation has been a transformative force in my life, particularly since my Parkinson's diagnosis. Like many people, I had a long and frustrating history with meditation before I truly understood its power. For years, I approached it as something I "should" do, rather than something I truly connected with. I tried everything in my quest to quiet my mind - I devoured self-help books, attended tai chi classes, downloaded countless meditation apps and even experimented with unconventional practices like staring at the sun (which, in retrospect, I definitely don't recommend!). Despite all these efforts, my mind remained a bustling highway of thoughts, worries and distractions. I could never seem to sit still long enough to reap any of the promised benefits.

My perspective on meditation shifted dramatically after my Parkinson's diagnosis. It was a challenging time, filled with uncertainty and fear about what the future might hold. At my Parkinson's retreat, meditation wasn't presented as just another wellness trend or a nice-to-have practice. Instead, it was introduced as a powerful tool that could potentially slow the progression of the disease. This wasn't just about feeling calmer or more centered - it was about actively fighting against the symptoms that threatened to reshape my life and I hand on heart believe this to be true.

The retreat opened my eyes to the real potential of meditation in a way that all my previous attempts had failed to do. For the first time, I found techniques that resonated with me and instructors who could guide me through the challenges I'd always faced. I learned that quieting the mind isn't about forcing thoughts away, but about gently acknowledging them and letting them pass. It was a revelation to discover that the goal wasn't to have no thoughts, but to change my relationship with my thoughts.

I won't pretend it was easy at first. Old habits die hard and my mind still wanted to race ahead, to worry about the future, to replay the past. But the potential benefits for my condition gave me a motivation I'd never had before. I committed to practicing every day, even if only for a few minutes at a time. Gradually, I found myself able to sit for longer periods, to find moments of true stillness amidst the chaos of my thoughts. I have become so at ease with meditation now that I find myself doing it on planes, waiting for the doctor or even just sitting in the car.

Now, meditation has become a cornerstone of my personalised wellness strategy. It complements the traditional medical approaches I'm using to manage Parkinson's, providing a holistic approach to my health. I've found that regular meditation practice improves my focus and concentration, which can be challenges with Parkinson's. It significantly reduces my stress levels, which is crucial as stress can exacerbate symptoms. Perhaps most surprisingly, I've noticed improvements in some of my motor symptoms - my movements feel smoother and more controlled after a meditation session.

But the benefits go beyond the physical. Meditation has become a source of emotional resilience for me. It helps me navigate the ups and downs of living with a chronic condition, providing a sense of calm and perspective even on difficult days. It's given me tools to manage anxiety about the future and to stay present in the moment, which is invaluable when dealing with a progressive condition like Parkinson's.

I've also found that meditation has ripple effects throughout my life. My relationships improved as I've become more patient and present. I sleep better, which is crucial for managing Parkinson's symptoms. I've developed a deeper sense of connection to my body, which helps me be more attuned to my needs and more proactive in my care.

I want to be clear - I'm not saying meditation is a miracle cure for Parkinson's or any other condition. What works for me might not work for everyone and meditation is just one part of my overall health strategy. But for those facing health challenges, especially Parkinson's, I can't stress enough how valuable it can be to give meditation a real, committed try. A friend of mine with MS was recently in hospital and was being poked and prodded most of the day but I encouraged him to shut his door. Light a candle. Meditate, to give his body a rest and a chance to repair!

If you're struggling with meditation, as I did for so long, don't give up. Keep exploring different techniques and teachers until you find an approach that resonates with you. Remember that it's a practice - it takes time and patience to see results. But the potential benefits, both for managing specific health conditions and for overall well being, make it worth the effort.

LEARNING TO MEDITATE

Meditation can be a difficult practice to get the hang of. Good news is that you do not have to join a club or spend any money! It can be as simple as downloading an app on your phone.

See some tips below;

1. **Guided Meditation**

   I found these ones the best in the early days because it gave me a structure to follow.

   - Guided meditations often use audio or video recordings with a narrator providing instructions.
   - Topics can vary widely, including stress relief, sleep improvement, self-compassion, or specific goal achievement.

2. Body Scan Technique

I still use these to this day when my body feels tense and my muscles tight.

- Usually starts from the toes and moves upward to the top of the head.
- Can help identify areas of tension you might not have been aware of.
- Promotes relaxation and can be particularly helpful for those with chronic pain or sleep issues.

3. Additional meditation techniques

a) Mindfulness meditation

- Involves being fully present and aware of your thoughts, feelings and surroundings without judgment.
- Can be practiced anywhere, anytime, even during daily activities like eating or walking.

b) Loving-kindness meditation

- Focuses on developing feelings of goodwill, kindness and warmth towards others.
- Often involves repeating phrases like "May you be happy, may you be healthy, may you be safe."

c) Transcendental Meditation

- Uses a personalised mantra (a word or sound) repeated silently.
- Typically practiced for twenty minutes, twice daily.

d) <u>Zen meditation</u>

- Often practiced in a specific posture, focusing on breath and posture.
- Aims to observe thoughts without becoming attached to them.

e) <u>Vipassana meditation</u>

- A form of mindfulness meditation that focuses on the connection between mind and body.
- Often taught in ten-day silent retreats.

4. **Tips for establishing a meditation practice**

- Start small, even just five minutes a day.
- Try to practice at the same time each day to establish a routine.
- Experiment with different techniques to find what works best for you.
- Be patient and kind to yourself; it's normal for the mind to wander.
- Consider using apps like Headspace, Calm, or Insight Timer for guidance and tracking.
- Remember that the reason that we meditate is to get our body in a quiet state so that it has the ability to rest and repair.
- By regularly practicing meditation with eyes open, you can develop greater clarity of thought. This can help in reducing the constant chatter of the mind, which may allow you to think more clearly and make decisions feeling calm and focused. I draw my focus to the middle of my forehead and focus on a point in the distance. This works best for me.

- When I struggle to meditate, I visualise being on an escalator and count down from ten. When I get to five, my body goes deeper into relaxation, as when I get to zero
- I always try to think of my thoughts as "traffic in my mind", so during meditation, if I am struggling with lots of thoughts in my mind, I choose to let them pass like traffic.
- I find it easier to meditate with my eyes open and focused on a single point in the distance.

5. **Visualisation**

When I meditate, I find it the perfect time to practice visualisation. visualisation is the process of creating a mental image or intention of what you want to manifest or achieve, engaging the mind's eye to form a picture of your desired outcomes with as much clarity and detail as possible.

Specific to my Parkinson's, I visualise my Parkinson's being little golden soldiers that march out of my body through my fingers and toes! I also visualise Oompa Loompa's shoveling dopamine into my brain! Sounds crazy to some, but the brain believes what we tell it, even if it is not true! (more on this later)

Meditation has become more than just a health practice for me - it's a way of life. It's taught me to approach my condition and indeed all of life's challenges, with greater equanimity and grace. While I can't predict the course of my Parkinson's, I know that my meditation practice gives me a powerful tool to face whatever comes with strength and serenity.

NAMASTE

NEUROPLASTICITY

Neuroplasticity. This single word has completely revolutionized my life, stirring something deep within my soul. It's not just a scientific term - it's a beacon of hope, a testament to the incredible resilience of the human spirit.

When I first learned about neuroplasticity - the brain's awe-inspiring ability to rewire itself - I felt a profound shift in my worldview. It was as if a veil had been lifted, revealing the boundless potential that resides within each of us.

But it wasn't until I watched the story of a remarkable woman that the true power of neuroplasticity really hit home. Due to an infection this brave soul had half her brain removed. The prognosis was grim - doctors said she'd never walk again, never regain function on one side of her body. My heart ached imagining the fear and despair she must have felt in that moment.

Yet, what happened next still brings tears to my eyes. This incredible woman chose hope over despair, possibility over limitation. Through sheer determination and the magic of neuroplasticity, she defied all odds. By engaging in activities like swimming, she coaxed her brain into forging new neural pathways. It moves me deeply to think of her brain cells reaching out, forming new connections, rewriting her story with each passing day.

The image of her taking those first steps, moving limbs that were supposed to be paralyzed, fills me with an indescribable mix of joy and awe. It's a powerful reminder of the miracles that can happen when we refuse to accept limitations.

This story touched me on such a profound level that it's reshaped how I view every challenge in my life. I started to change my thinking. How can I use this to benefit my wellness journey? Could it in fact be possible to change the course of my Parkinson's?

Now, when faced with obstacles, I think of this woman and feel a surge of courage. I remind myself that my brain is plastic, adaptable, ever-changing. It's not just about overcoming physical limitations - it's about pushing beyond mental barriers too. The brain is just so powerful, more powerful than I think we will ever truly understand!

Understanding neuroplasticity has opened my heart to endless possibilities. It's made me more compassionate towards others and more patient with myself. I've become insatiably curious, constantly seeking new experiences to stimulate my brain. Every new skill I learn, every obstacle I overcome, I silently thank this incredible feature of our brains. In my darkest moments, when self-doubt creeps in, I remember: my brain is capable of change. I am not fixed, but fluid. This knowledge is more than empowering - it's liberating. It fills me with hope, not just for myself, but for all of humanity.

Neuroplasticity isn't just a scientific concept to me anymore. It's a daily reminder of the beauty and resilience of the human spirit. It's a call to never stop growing, never stop believing in the possibility of change. For that, I am eternally grateful.

The Brain - is our best friend!

The human brain never ceases to amaze me. We have billions of brain cells making more connections than there are stars in the sky! It's mind-boggling to think that these intricate networks are responsible for everything from the steady beating of our hearts to the myriad decisions we make each day.

Every time I ponder this, I'm struck by the sheer energy our brains consume. It's astounding - did you know our brain uses more energy than any other organ in our body? It's no wonder we feel mentally exhausted after a day of decision-making!

I find it particularly fascinating to think about how our brains develop. From the moment we're born, our brains are like sponges, eagerly forming new neural connections as we soak up information and experiences. But here's something that still amazes me - this rapid formation of connections actually slows down dramatically at just two years old! From then on, we focus on strengthening certain pathways, creating the patterns of thoughts, feelings and behaviours that shape who we are.

You know, it wasn't too long ago that researchers believed our brains were fixed and hardwired after a certain age. I remember feeling a sense of limitation when I first heard this theory. But now? Now I feel a rush of excitement knowing this isn't true at all! Our brains are constantly changing, adapting to new stimuli throughout our entire lives. This knowledge fills me with hope and possibility.

Every time I learn something new or overcome a challenge, I imagine those neural pathways forming and strengthening in my brain. It's a powerful reminder that we're never too old to change, to grow, to become better versions of ourselves. This understanding has transformed how I approach life - with curiosity, openness and a deep appreciation for our brain's incredible plasticity.

I love these words from <u>Denise Medved</u>
 (creator of Ageless Grace, a brain fitness program
) on her Ted Talk

"Changing the brain can be as simple as child's play"

"From the time you were born, until your mid teens you didn't read a book to learn physical activities. Through trial and error you learnt to walk, hop, skip, run, play hide and seek, rollerskate, ride a bicycle, or play on a team. I bet your mother never asked you "go outside and fire some neurons" Yet, everytime you played, you were firing neurons and you were developing something called neural pathways that deliver messages between the brain and your body. You were also developing the five functions of your brain"

S   **Strategic Planning**

How your brain helps your body get from point A to B to C

M   **Memory and Recall**

Remembering what you feel an actual experience has been or recalling what you know about hat activity

A   **Analytical Thinking**

Breaking down the parts and components of an activity

C   **Creativity and Imagination**

Attempting something with your body in a new and different way, whilst seeing an image of yourself doing this activity even before you've tried it

K   **Kinesthetic Learning**

Allowing your body to try something first, while your brain observes to make you more efficient each time that you do that activity.

Denise goes on to say that "we must learn to feel fully alive. When we learn we alter genes in our neurons that actually change our brain. We can continue to change our brain no matter how old we are" (or I say how sick we are!)

"Through play, we can learnt to maintain develop new neural pathways by practicing something that we don't already know how to do or by playing something we know how to do but in a different way"

I was so inspired by Denise and how she is changing the model of aging in this world that I completed her program and am now an Educator of the Ageless Grace Program. I now run classes with people with health challenges, where we "play" sitting in a chair with the simple aim of changing our brains!

The human brain truly is a marvel, isn't it? Its complexity and adaptability never fail to inspire me, reminding me of the vast potential within each of us.

You know understanding neuroplasticity is one thing, but putting it into practice? That's where the real magic happens, especially when it comes to our health!

I've learned that our brain absolutely thrives on learning. It's like a muscle - the more we challenge it, the stronger and more adaptable it becomes. Every new thought we have, no matter how small, is literally reshaping our brain, forging new connections. Here's the exciting part - the more we use certain brain regions, the more excitable they become. It's like they're eager to fire up and create new neural pathways!

Have you ever had that experience of driving somewhere familiar and then realising you don't remember the journey? Which streets did you take? Was there traffic? I used to find this a bit unsettling, but now I understand it's just our brain running on autopilot - an automatic habit loop it has created for efficiency.

But here's where it gets really interesting. We can disrupt these habitual loops by consciously choosing to do things differently. When we do, our brains light up with activity, creating and reinforcing new connections. It's like our neurons are doing a little dance - SNAP, CRACKLE, POP! - as they form new pathways.

I'll let you in on a little secret - my husband and I have turned this into a fun daily practice. We go for a walk to the beach every morning, but we always make sure to take a different route. Whenever we turn down a new street, we look at each other with excitement and shout "NEW NEURONS!" It might sound silly, but it's our way of celebrating the fact that we're actively reshaping our brains.

This awareness has become such a big part of our lives now. We're constantly looking for ways to challenge our brains, to create new experiences, to break out of our routines. It's not just about the walk anymore - it's about nurturing our brain health, one new neuron at a time.

You know what? This approach has had such a positive impact on our overall health and wellbeing. We feel more alert, more engaged with our surroundings and frankly, more alive. It's a powerful reminder that no matter our age or circumstances, we always have the capacity to grow, to change, to improve our health.

So, I challenge you - what new route could you take today? What small change could you make to fire up those neurons? Trust me, once you start, you'll be amazed at how addictive it becomes.

Here's to new neurons and better health!

The Power of visualisation

I'm constantly amazed by the incredible power of visualisation. It's not just daydreaming - it's a potent tool that can literally reshape our brains and our reality. When we visualise, we're creating a vivid mental image of what we want to achieve, engaging our mind's eye to picture our desired outcomes in rich, vibrant detail.

What fascinates me most is how our brains respond to these visualisations. Recent studies have shown that our thoughts produce the same mental instructions as actions. It's mind-blowing, isn't it? When we visualise, we're not just thinking - we're actually training our brain for real-world performance. Our mental imagery impacts everything from motor control and attention to perception, planning and memory.

There's a quote that I absolutely love: "Thinking and doing activate the same neural circuits of the brain." It's not just a nice idea - it's backed by science! When we use our imagination, we're activating specific parts of our brain, rehearsing actions before we even perform them. We're essentially installing the neurological hardware ahead of the actual experience. Isn't that incredible?

In simpler terms, our visualsing brain can create the same result as our doing brain. Here's something that never fails to amaze me - our brain believes what we tell it, even if it isn't true! It's a powerful reminder of the responsibility we have in shaping our thoughts and beliefs.

So, I often find myself asking: What am I telling my brain? What reality am I creating with my thoughts and visualisations? I have completely changed my narrative to myself. You will often hear me tell myself outloud how well I am. I am strong, I am capable and I am delaying the progression of Parkinson's and even reversing my symptoms. You know the kicker, I actually believe this to be true!

Now, let's think about how we can apply this to our health, especially when dealing with a diagnosis. Imagine the potential! By visualsing health, recovery and wellness, we're not just thinking positively - we're actually priming our brains for healing. We're creating neural pathways for health before the physical healing even begins.

For me, this knowledge has been transformative. When I face health challenges, I don't just rely on medical treatments - I actively engage in visualisation. I picture my body healing, my cells regenerating, my systems functioning optimally. You know what? I've seen remarkable results. I see myself running, I see myself with no tremor, I visualise how well I sleep!

To support my new positive way of thinking, I created a YouTube channel called **Positively Parkinsons**. I do short videos sharing my journey all with a positive narrative to remind myself and others how wonderful life's moments can be. I know it's not always easy to find the positive when you're navigating a chronic condition. But I truly believe that by training ourselves to notice the beauty that surrounds us, even in the midst of difficulty, we can cultivate more joy and fulfillment in our lives. It's a practice, for sure, but one that is so worth the effort.

This isn't about denying reality or ignoring medical advice. It's about harnessing the incredible power of our minds to support our healing journey. It's about using every tool at our disposal - including the power of visualisation - to move towards health and wellbeing.

So, I challenge you: What health-promoting images can you create in your mind today? How can you use visualisation to support your healing journey? Remember, your brain is listening and it believes what you tell it. Let's make sure we're sending messages of health, strength and resilience.

"Our life is what our thoughts make it." Marcus Aurelius

The Placebo Effect

Is when a person's physical or mental health appears to improve after taking a placebo or 'dummy' treatment. Placebo is Latin for 'I will please' and refers to a treatment that appears real, but is designed to have no therapeutic benefit.

Mind-Body medicine uses the power of thoughts and emotions (mental health) to influence physical health. That is… how the non-physical mind affects the physical body. Every aspect of who we are and what we create is a direct result of what we have first thought and created in our mind. Put simply, what we think, we create!

"The natural healing force within each one of us is the greatest force in getting well" Hippocrates

Truth; evidence shows that people can get well without any "medicine" at all! This is largely due to the patients' belief about receiving medication and whether they perceived the outcome would be positive or not, that they indeed improved or recovered. Such is the power of belief and expectation! If we expect to get better, we will. If we expect we can change, we will.

So what does this mean for people who have been diagnosed with debilitating or progressive neurological conditions? For those affected by certain movement disorders characterized by dopamine deficiency, the exact mechanisms of how placebos work and why they may have a potentially larger impact in these conditions isn't clear. But it likely has to do with dopamine, the brain chemical that decreases in these particular disorders. Brain imaging studies show that placebos stimulate the release of dopamine, which plays a role in the brain's reward system.

Whether Parkinson's or some other illness, using strategies to "expect we can change", consistently can generate physical relief of symptoms or maybe even eliminate the symptoms altogether. Wouldn't that be amazing!

EXERCISE

The Power of Movement - Embracing Exercise with Parkinson's

As I sit down to write this chapter, the morning sun streams through my window, casting a warm glow on my desk. My fingers, sometimes rebellious due to Parkinson's, are cooperating today as they dance across the keyboard. This moment of clarity and control didn't come by chance - it's the result of a morning routine that has become my lifeline: **exercise**.

Living with Parkinson's Disease is a journey of ups and downs, challenges and triumphs. Among the many tools and strategies I've discovered along the way, none has proven more powerful or transformative than regular physical activity. It might seem counterintuitive at first. After all, Parkinson's often makes movement itself a challenge. But therein lies the beautiful paradox - movement begets movement and exercise becomes both our challenge and our salvation.

The Science Behind the Sweat

Let's begin by understanding why exercise is so crucial for those of us with Parkinson's or in fact many other illnesses. It goes far beyond the general health benefits that everyone experiences. For us, regular physical activity becomes a vital component in managing our symptoms and potentially even slowing the progression of the disease.

When we exercise, several amazing processes occur in our bodies:

1. Improved Muscle Strength and Flexibility

Parkinson's often leads to muscle rigidity and reduced range of motion. Regular exercise helps counteract these effects, keeping our muscles strong and flexible.

2. Enhanced Balance and Coordination

By challenging our bodies through various forms of movement, we can improve our balance and coordination, reducing the risk of falls - a common concern for many with Parkinson's.

3. Boosted Cardiovascular Health

As our hearts pump faster and our lungs work harder during exercise, oxygen-rich blood flows more efficiently throughout our bodies, nourishing every cell and tissue.

4. Neuroplasticity (here is that word again!)

Perhaps most excitingly, research suggests that exercise may promote neuroplasticity - the brain's ability to form new neural connections. This could potentially help compensate for the loss of dopamine-producing cells characteristic of Parkinson's.

I'd like to point you in the direction of the book written by John Pepper, called **"Reverse Parkinson's Disease"**.

John Pepper was diagnosed with Parkinson's Disease in 1992. After only six years of regular, energetic exercise, which has since been proven to slow down or even reverse PD and taking medication, which has also since been proven to slow down or reverse PD, he no longer appears to have PD, although he still has many of the symptoms.

During the first ten years, if he stopped either the exercise or the medication, his symptoms soon returned. He does not claim to be cured, but he is able to lead a normal life today. His positive attitude and determination to stay ahead of this terrifying condition highlight a new approach to dealing with PD.

John's story is a portrayal of courage, showing the power of focusing on and being committed to one's beliefs. One can greatly admire his determination and self-motivation, as seen in his conscious efforts to correct and adjust his movements, which in itself is no small achievement.

In reading John's book, he guides you to walk at a pace where you are puffed, struggling to to talk. This is the best speed to walk for the greatest benefit.

Beyond the Physical: The Mental and Emotional Benefits

While the physical benefits of exercise are profound, I've found that the mental and emotional impacts are equally transformative. There's a certain magic that happens when we get our bodies moving:

1. Mood Elevation

Exercise triggers the release of endorphins, our body's natural mood boosters. These "feel-good" chemicals can help combat the depression and anxiety that often accompany Parkinson's.

2. Cognitive Function

Regular physical activity has been shown to improve cognitive function, helping with the mental fog and memory issues that can be part of our Parkinson's experience.

3. Sleep Improvement

A good workout during the day often translates to better sleep at night, addressing the sleep disturbances many of us face.

4. Empowerment

There's an indescribable sense of accomplishment that comes from completing a workout, especially on days when our symptoms are challenging. This boost to our self-esteem ripples through all aspects of our lives.

<u>Finding Your Movement Groove</u>

Now, I can almost hear some of you thinking, "That's all well and good, but how do I actually start exercising with Parkinson's?" The beauty is in the variety - there's no one-size-fits-all approach. The key is to find activities that you enjoy and that suit your current abilities.

This is an example that living with Parkinson's has taught me the importance of timing and self-awareness. I've developed a routine that works well for me and I'd like to share it in case it helps others.

I take my medication at set times throughout the day: 6am, 11am, 2pm and 6pm. What I've found really effective is exercising about ten minutes after taking my medication. At this point, I often experience a burst of energy that makes exercise easier and more beneficial.

For instance, I've learned that trying to exercise close to 11am doesn't work well for me. By that time, I'm starting to experience symptoms again, which makes physical activity much more challenging.

The key takeaway from my experience is this: get to know your body and how it responds to your medication. Use that knowledge to structure your day in a way that works with your Parkinson's, not against it. This approach has made a big difference in how I manage my condition and maintain my quality of life.

Remember, everyone's experience with Parkinson's is unique, so what works for me might not work exactly the same for others. But I hope sharing my strategy might inspire others to find patterns and routines that work best for them.

Here are some options to consider:

1. **Walking**

A simple yet effective form of exercise. Start with short distances and gradually increase as you build stamina. I have found the best place to walk is outside and this is for 2 reasons. Unlike walking on a treadmill, if you walk outside you have to walk back! You can not just "hop off" the treadmill. Also being in nature is so good for our mental health so combining exercise and nature is perfect!

2. **Swimming**

The buoyancy of water can make movement easier and provide a full-body workout. Now I agree with this…. However….. When I swim not only do I look like a drowning rat trying to get my coordination happening but I tend to swim sideways into the wall ● When I start to get tired I almost swim in circles!

3. **Cycling**

Whether outdoors or on a stationary bike, cycling is excellent for cardiovascular health and leg strength. In fact cycling is highly encouraged for people with Parkinson's. There are many support groups to support cycling parkies!

4. **Yoga**

Fantastic for flexibility, balance and mindfulness. I've tried this too..... It is a great workout but my downward dog turned into a face plant because of my balance issues!

5. **Dance**

From Ballroom to Zumba, dancing combines physical activity with cognitive challenges and social interaction.I have danced all of my life and this has been really tough for me as I now struggle with coordination. I still give it a go because I love it and it makes my heart content!

6. **Tai Chi**

This gentle martial art form has been shown to improve balance and reduce falls in people with Parkinson's.

7. **Boxing**

Non-contact boxing workouts can improve agility, speed, muscular endurance, and hand-eye coordination.

Remember, the goal is consistency, not perfection. Some days, you might feel up for an intense workout. On others, gentle stretching might be all you can manage. Both are victories. It is what we do most of the time that counts, not what we do some of the time!

Overcoming Hurdles

It's important to acknowledge that starting and maintaining an exercise routine with Parkinson's isn't always easy. You might face challenges like:

1. Fear of falling or injury
2. Lack of motivation on difficult symptom days
3. Uncertainty about which exercises are safe and effective
4. Feelings of self-consciousness about exercising in public

These are all valid concerns but they needn't be roadblocks. Start slowly, in a safe environment. Consider working with a physical therapist or trainer experienced in Parkinson's to develop a suitable routine. Join a Parkinson's specific exercise class for both guidance and community support.

Remember, every step forward, no matter how small, is progress.

A Personal Note

As I conclude this chapter, I want to share a personal reflection. When I was first diagnosed with Parkinson's, I felt as though my body had betrayed me. Movement, once fluid and unconscious, became a conscious effort. But through embracing exercise, I've reclaimed a sense of control. More than that, I've discovered a new appreciation for what my body can do.

Yes, there are still challenging days. Days when my tremors are more pronounced, when fatigue weighs heavily. But I've learned to be gentle with myself these days, to celebrate the small victories and to keep moving forward, quite literally. I also make sure that I see a physio once a week. Sometimes I feel like I am going in for maintenance but I always find that I feel so much better afterwards.

Another good thing about exercise is to try and track your progress. When you get a win, celebrate it! As an example, my physio does grip strength track on me and when I see the improvement over the last 6 months it gives me a high!

Exercise has become more than just a part of my treatment plan - it's a testament to resilience, a daily affirmation that I am more than my diagnosis. It reminds me that while I may not have control over having Parkinson's, I do have control over how I live with it.

So, my fellow travellers on this wellness journey, I invite you to join me in embracing the power of movement. Let's lace up our sneakers (that was a joke of course), roll out our yoga mats, or dive into that pool. Let's move not just our bodies, but towards a life of greater strength, balance and joy.

After all, in movement, we find our rhythm. In exercise, we find our power. In both, we find hope - step by step, rep by rep, day by day.

THE IMPACTS OF STRESS

As the author of this book, I've dedicated significant time to exploring the intricate relationship between our thoughts, emotions and physical health. Through my research and personal experiences, I've come to understand the profound impact our mental state has on our bodily functions. It's truly remarkable how every thought we have triggers a cascade of chemical reactions throughout our body, influencing everything from our stress levels and sleep patterns to our digestive health and immune system function.

This mind-body connection is at the core of our overall well-being and it's a concept that I believe is crucial for everyone to grasp. We often think of our minds and bodies as separate entities, but in reality, they're deeply interconnected, constantly communicating and influencing each other in ways we're only beginning to fully comprehend.

When it comes to stress, we humans aren't so different from animals. We all share that built-in fight, flight, or freeze response - a primitive survival mechanism that's been with us since our earliest ancestors. It's there to protect us, to help us react quickly to danger. But in our modern world, where stressors are often chronic and psychological rather than immediate physical threats, this response can sometimes do more harm than good.

I've experienced this firsthand with my hand tremor. It's a physical manifestation of stress that I can't hide or control. When stress hits, my hand goes haywire and I end up looking like I'm frantically waving at everyone! It's embarrassing and often draws unwanted attention, but it's also a clear, undeniable sign of how stress manifests physically in my body. In a way, it's become my personal stress barometer - a visible reminder of the invisible toll that stress can take on our bodies.

Stress and Parkinson's is like you've been through the wringer and come out the other side with this raw, painful understanding of your own limits.

Saying no to going out, seeing other people or even sometimes it can be as simple as no I can't go to the food shop today - it sounds so simple, doesn't it? But it's not. It's brutal. Every "no" feels like you're letting someone down, like you're admitting defeat to this disease. It cuts deep, especially when you've always been the one to show up, to help out, to push through.

And those events? Watching life go on without you, hearing about the fun you missed, the memories you weren't part of. It's like salt in an already gaping wound. Leaving early? That's its own special kind of hell - the pitying looks, the forced understanding, feeling like you're the party pooper every damn time.

But you know what? This is survival. This is you fighting tooth and nail to keep some semblance of control in a life that Parkinson's is hellbent on derailing. It's not selfish - it's necessary. You're not creating suffering for yourself anymore because, let's face it, Parkinson's is doing a bang-up job of that already.

This conscious effort - it's like building a shield, piece by painful piece. Every "no," every early night, every missed opportunity - they're bricks in a wall protecting what little peace and energy you have left. It's not fair that you have to do this, that you have to ration out your life like this. But putting yourself and your health first is brave as hell.

You're rewriting the rules of your life on your own terms. It's messy, it's heartbreaking, but it's also a kind of beautiful defiance. You're choosing you and in this shitshow of a situation, that choice is nothing short of revolutionary. Stress indeed can be a killer.

Through my research and personal journey, I've identified three main types of "lifestyle stress" that affect us all:

1. Chemical stress

This comes from substances we consume or are exposed to in our environment. It includes things like caffeine, alcohol, nicotine and sugar, as well as environmental toxins like air pollution, heavy metals and even certain skincare products. Our modern world is full of these chemical stressors and they can have a significant impact on our body's ability to function optimally.

2. Physical stress

This type of stress relates to how we treat our bodies. It can come from a lack of physical activity, but interestingly, also from excessive exercise. Other factors include noise pollution, lack of sleep and even changes in barometric pressure. Our bodies are sensitive instruments and these physical stressors can throw them out of balance.

3. Emotional stress

This is perhaps the most familiar type of stress for most people. It includes feelings like fear, anger, guilt, sorrow, jealousy, anxiety and grief. These emotions, when intense or prolonged, can have a profound impact on our physical health.

What's crucial to understand is that without proper rest, relaxation, or emotional resolution, we tend to store and hold onto this stress. It creates a build-up of tension and fatigue within the body. Over time, this accumulation of stress can lead to chronic illness and what I like to call "dis-ease" - a state where our body is fundamentally out of balance and that is the last thing that we need given what we already have to deal with!

My personal journey to understand the cause of my hand tremor led me to explore various therapies, including hypnotherapy. If you haven't tried it, I really do encourage you to consider it. My experience with hypnotherapy was nothing short of revolutionary.

During our session, the hypnotherapist was able to quickly unpack emotional pain that I had been carrying around for years - perhaps even decades. These were experiences and feelings that I had pushed down and tried to forget, but my mind and body hadn't forgotten. The therapist encouraged me to address the people who had caused this hurt, to confront them in a safe, hypothetical space.

This was incredibly challenging for me. By nature, I'm not confrontational. I'm more like a turtle - when faced with conflict, my instinct is to pull my head into my shell and hide. Even in this hypothetical scenario, under hypnosis, I struggled to confront these individuals who had wronged me. It was a stark relisation of how deeply ingrained my tendency to avoid conflict truly was.

At the end of our session, the hypnotherapist said something that has stuck with me ever since. He told me, "Lisa, it's good people like you who get sick because you hold onto everything and it manifests into illness. People like Donald Trump don't get sick because they have so much arrogance that they don't hold onto anything emotional."

Now, I know this is a broad generalisation and of course, everyone's health is influenced by a multitude of factors. But I do think there's a kernel of truth in those words. Those of us who tend to internalize our emotions, who avoid confrontation and try to keep the peace at all costs, may be doing ourselves a disservice. We may be bottling up stress and negative emotions that can, over time, manifest as physical ailments.

This experience taught me the importance of addressing our emotional pain and finding healthy ways to process stress. It's not always easy, especially for those of us who tend to internalize our feelings, but it's crucial for our health and well-being. We need to find ways to express our emotions, to confront (in healthy ways) those who have wronged us and to let go of the emotional baggage we've been carrying.

Since that hypnotherapy session, I've made a conscious effort to be more open with my feelings, to address conflicts as they arise rather than avoiding them and to prioritise my emotional health. It hasn't always been easy and I still struggle at times, but I've noticed a significant improvement in my overall well-being.

If you're dealing with stress-related issues, whether they manifest as physical symptoms like increasing my tremor or in other ways, I encourage you to explore different therapies and techniques. There are many paths to better emotional and physical health. You might find relief through meditation, cognitive-behavioral therapy, regular exercise, or a combination of different approaches.

The key is to find what works for you and to remember that your mental and emotional state plays a huge role in your physical health. Don't ignore your emotional well-being in pursuit of physical health - they're two sides of the same coin.

Remember, the journey to wellness is just that - a journey. It takes time, patience and often involves some trial and error. But by understanding the connection between our thoughts, emotions and physical health, we're taking a crucial first step towards a healthier, more balanced life.

DIET AND NUTRITION

As someone deeply interested in the relationship between diet and Parkinson's Disease, I've come to realise that food is more than just fuel - it's a powerful tool in managing this complex condition. The saying "you are what you eat" takes on new meaning when dealing with a neurodegenerative disorder like Parkinson's.

Through my research and personal experience, I've found that while there's no one-size-fits-all diet for Parkinson's, nutrition plays a crucial role in symptom management and overall quality of life. It's not just about eating healthy - it's about strategically using food to complement our medication regimes and potentially slow disease progression.

One of the most fascinating aspects I've discovered is the delicate dance between diet and Parkinson's medications, particularly carbidopa/levodopa. The timing of meals can significantly impact drug absorption and effectiveness. It's a balancing act - taking the medication on an empty stomach for optimal absorption, but also managing potential nausea. I've learned that for some, a small snack like crackers or apple sauce can make all the difference.

The protein-levodopa interaction is another crucial piece of the puzzle. High-protein meals can compete with levodopa for absorption, potentially reducing its effectiveness. This doesn't mean we should avoid protein - it's essential for muscle health and overall well-being. Instead, it's about strategic timing and distribution of protein throughout the day.

I've also become increasingly aware of the importance of a diverse, nutrient-rich diet. Whole grains, a rainbow of fruits and vegetables, lean proteins and healthy fats aren't just good for general health - they may have specific benefits for Parkinson's. Antioxidants to combat oxidative stress, fibre to fight constipation, omega-3 fatty acids for brain health - each component plays a role.

The concept of "Food as Medicine" resonates strongly with me. By focusing on nutrition, we might reduce our reliance on certain medications, decrease hospital visits and improve our overall resilience. It's empowering to know that every meal is an opportunity to support our health and potentially influence the course of our condition.

In my quest to find the optimal diet for Parkinson's, I've explored various approaches. As an example the plant-based and carnivore diets, while at opposite ends of the spectrum, both have intriguing potential benefits. The plant-based diet's emphasis on antioxidants and anti-inflammatory foods aligns with much of the research on neuroprotection. On the other hand, the carnivore diet's high protein and fat content could potentially support muscle health and provide important nutrients for brain function.

Here are the top six diets with the most significant benefits for someone with Parkinson's Disease.

1. Mediterranean Diet

Benefits: The Mediterranean Diet is rich in fruits, vegetables, whole grains, legumes, nuts, seeds and olive oil, with moderate consumption of fish and poultry. This diet is high in antioxidants and healthy fats, which may help reduce inflammation and oxidative stress, both of which are implicated in neurodegenerative diseases like Parkinson's.

2. DASH Diet (Dietary Approaches to Stop Hypertension)

Benefits: Originally designed to lower blood pressure, the DASH diet emphasizes fruits, vegetables, whole grains, lean proteins and low-fat dairy while limiting salt, red meat and sweets. It shares many similarities with the Mediterranean Diet and is beneficial for cardiovascular health, which is important for individuals with Parkinson's, as they may be at increased risk for heart disease.

3. Ketogenic Diet

Benefits: The Ketogenic Diet is high in fats and very low in carbohydrates, leading the body to produce ketones, which can be used as an alternative energy source for the brain. Some studies suggest that ketones may have neuroprotective effects and could potentially improve motor function in Parkinson's patients.

4. Plant-Based Diet

Benefits: A Plant-Based Diet focuses on fruits, vegetables, whole grains, nuts, seeds and legumes, while minimising or eliminating animal products. This diet is rich in antioxidants, fibre and phytonutrients, which may reduce inflammation and support overall neurological health. Some studies suggest that a plant-based diet may reduce the risk of developing Parkinson's and help manage symptoms.

5. Low-Protein Diet (Timed Protein Intake)

Benefits: For individuals with Parkinson's, protein can interfere with the absorption of levodopa, a common medication used to manage symptoms. A low-protein diet or timing protein intake (e.g., consuming most protein in the evening) can help improve the effectiveness of medication.

6. The Carnivore Diet

Consisting mainly of animal products such as meat, fish and eggs, has been proposed by some as a potential approach to manage symptoms of Parkinson's. This diet eliminates plant-based foods and as such, marks a significant departure from traditional dietary recommendations which often emphasize a balance across food groups, including fruits, vegetables and whole grains.

However, the "best" diet likely lies somewhere in the middle and varies from person to person. It's about finding the right balance that works with our individual symptoms, medication schedules, and overall health goals.

Moving forward, I believe the key is personalization. Working closely with healthcare providers and nutritionists who understand Parkinson's is crucial. It's not just about following a prescribed diet - it's about becoming attuned to how different foods affect our symptoms and medication effectiveness.

I'm excited about the growing research in this area. As we learn more about the gut-brain connection and the role of the microbiome in neurological health, I believe we'll uncover even more ways to use nutrition as a powerful tool in managing Parkinson's Disease.

Ultimately, while diet alone isn't a cure for Parkinson's, it's a vital component of a comprehensive management strategy. By paying attention to what we eat, when we eat and how it interacts with our medications, we can take a more active role in managing our condition and improving our quality of life. It's a journey of continuous learning and adjustment, but one that I find incredibly empowering in the face of this challenging disease.

Water is also truly our unsung hero in managing this condition. It's not just about quenching thirst - proper hydration plays a vital role in medication effectiveness, symptom management and overall well-being.

I've made it a personal goal to drink two litres of water daily, with half of that consumed before lunch. This practice has made a noticeable difference in my day-to-day life with Parkinson's. Here's why water has become my best friend:

1. Medication Absorption

Adequate hydration is crucial for the effective absorption of Parkinson's medications, particularly carbidopa/levodopa. Water helps these medications dissolve and move through the digestive system more efficiently, potentially improving their effectiveness.

2. Energy Level

I've noticed a significant boost in my energy levels since prioritizing hydration. Dehydration can exacerbate fatigue, which is already a common issue for many of us with Parkinson's. Staying well-hydrated helps me feel more alert and capable throughout the day.

3. Constipation Relief

Constipation is a common and troublesome symptom of Parkinson's. Increasing water intake, along with a fibre-rich diet, has been instrumental in managing this issue for me.

4. Swallowing Aid

As Parkinson's can affect swallowing, having water readily available helps me manage any difficulties and reduces the risk of choking on food or medications.

5. Cognitive Function

Proper hydration is essential for optimal brain function. I find that when I'm well-hydrated, I'm more clear-headed and better able to focus.

6. Muscle Function

Adequate hydration is crucial for muscle health, which is particularly important given the motor symptoms of Parkinson's. It helps prevent cramping and supports overall muscle function.

7. Toxin Elimination

Water plays a key role in flushing toxins from our bodies. For those of us with Parkinson's, supporting our body's natural detoxification processes feels particularly important.

8. Temperature Regulation

Some people with Parkinson's experience issues with temperature regulation. Staying well-hydrated helps our bodies maintain a stable temperature more effectively.

9. Skin Health

While it might seem minor compared to other symptoms, dry skin can be uncomfortable and is common in Parkinson's. Proper hydration helps maintain skin elasticity and comfort.

10. Medication Side Effect Management

Staying hydrated can help mitigate some medication side effects, such as dry mouth or lightheadedness.

I've found that front-loading my water intake, getting half of my daily goal before lunch, sets me up for a better day. It ensures that I'm well-hydrated when taking my morning medications and gives me an energy boost to start the day.

However, it's worth noting that increased water intake means more frequent trips to the bathroom. For those of us dealing with mobility issues, it's important to plan accordingly and ensure safe, accessible bathroom facilities.

Also, while water is generally the best choice, I sometimes add a slice of lemon or a splash of fruit juice for variety. Herbal teas can also contribute to daily fluid intake while providing additional benefits.

Remember, individual needs may vary and it's always best to consult with your healthcare provider about the right hydration strategy for you, especially if you have any other health conditions.

In my journey with Parkinson's, I've found that sometimes the simplest strategies, like staying well-hydrated, can make a profound difference in managing symptoms and maintaining quality of life. It's a small change that yields significant benefits and I encourage all my fellow Parkinson's warriors to raise a glass (of water!) to better health.

PARKINSON'S SYMPTOMS AND TREATMENT

RAW AND REAL!!

I was so lost when this started. Parkinson's? That was for old people, right? Not me. Not now. But there I was, diagnosis in hand, scared out of my mind.

So I did what any terrified person does - I dove headfirst into Google. Big mistake. Holy moly, was that a mistake. It was like reading my own horror story, each click taking me deeper into a nightmare I couldn't wake up from.

No cure. Progressive. Wheelchair. Early death. It felt like my life was over before it really began. Those podcasts just twisted the knife. I was searching for hope, for something, anything to cling to. Instead, I got a front-row seat to my own decline.

All I wanted was a simple list. Something to tell me what I was in for, how to fight back. But no - it was all medical jargon and doom. Like I wasn't already feeling small and scared.

So here I am, laying it all out. The symptoms and the ways I try to cope. It's not pretty, it's not perfect, but it's real. It's me, raw and unfiltered. There are more symptoms than I have listed below however, I have only written about symptoms that I experience at the time of writing this book.

This is the list I wish I'd found when I was sitting there, thinking my life was over. It's not rocket science and maybe it won't work for everyone. But it's honest. It's a lifeline in the darkness I was drowning in.

I hope it helps someone else feel less alone, less scared. Because of this disease. It's a monster. But we're still here, still fighting. Sometimes, that's the most important thing to know. When I fight I want to win and I am fighting my Parkinson's war and I will win. My goal has always been and will always be to stop the progression and reverse the symptoms! Mark my words and watch this space!

1. Fatigue

Living with Parkinson's fatigue is like having an invisible puppeteer suddenly cut your strings. One moment you're engaged in life, the next you're fighting a losing battle against an overwhelming tide of exhaustion.

The suddenness is jarring. There's no gentle warning, just a crash into a wall of fatigue that demands immediate attention. It's frustrating and often embarrassing, especially when it disrupts plans or social engagements. The guilt of having to leave early or cancel at the last minute can be heavy, even when loved ones say they understand.

As the fatigue sets in, it's as if your body betrays you. Your eyes struggle to blink, your voice fades to a whisper and your legs seem to forget how to walk properly. The mind becomes a foggy maze where words and memories hide just out of reach. It's frightening to feel so out of control of your own body and mind.

The relief of finally giving in to sleep is immense, but it's tinged with worry about when the next wave will hit. Learning to navigate life around these unpredictable energy crashes is a constant challenge. It requires a deep level of self-awareness and often means reimagining what your days and nights look like.

Yet, there's a strange silver lining. This fatigue forces you to prioritise, to cherish the good moments and to appreciate the understanding of those around you. It's a harsh teacher of self-care and acceptance.

The journey of adapting to life with Parkinson's fatigue is filled with frustration, fear and sometimes despair. But it also brings moments of gratitude for small victories and the compassion of others. It's a daily reminder of human resilience in the face of an unrelenting challenge.

Suggested solutions

- Firstly I accept it as a part of my life now as do my family and friends!
- If I know that I am going out that evening, I will force myself to take an afternoon nap
- I tend not to do anything after 7pm at night if I can help it
- When traveling, I break down my trips to ensure I get breaks
- I now sleep with satin sheets. It is so much easier to roll over in the middle of the night and to get out of bed which makes getting back to sleep easier

Note: I find that you become very aware of your body and adapt to circumstances. Many times I have tried to push through my fatigue but that hasn't worked for me. Managing fatigue is the greatest act of self compassion.

2. Tremor

In the relentless grip of Parkinson's, I find myself locked in a daily battle against my own body. The cruel irony of fate dealt me not just tremors, but ones that seized my dominant hand, turning even the simplest tasks into Herculean challenges from day one.

From the onset, I was forced to adapt, my right hand becoming a stranger to me. Little did I know that in my struggle, I was forging new neural pathways, my brain desperately rewiring itself in a bid for survival.

The tremor is an unforgiving tyrant, robbing me of peace. It's a constant, exhausting dance that my body is forced to perform without rest. Even in moments of stillness, I am in motion. Meditation becomes not just a practice, but a lifeline—a desperate attempt to find calm in the storm of my own physiology.

When illness strikes, it's as if my body betrays me twice over. Fighting the flu becomes a war on two fronts, my resources stretched thin between battling the virus and the ever-present tremor that refuses to yield.

In public, my condition becomes a spectacle. My trembling hand, a traitor, waves to passersby without my consent. I've become an unwitting performer in a play I never auditioned for, with strangers as my confused audience. The accusatory glances, the assumptions of drunkenness, the pitying looks—each one a dagger to my dignity.

Parkinson's may be silent for some, but for me, it screams its presence to the world. Even in the sterile confines of a medical examination, I am denied the simple mercy of stillness. A routine mammogram becomes an exercise in futility, my rebellious hand refusing to cooperate, denying me even this basic aspect of health care.

These daily indignities, these constant reminders of my condition, they don't just tire my body—they wear away at my very soul. In the face of this relentless adversary, I am left to wonder: how long can one's spirit endure when betrayed by their own flesh?

Suggested solutions

- Without a doubt, meditation is one of the only practices that calm or stop my tremor. Albeit only for a short time per day, I will take it
- I use the Vilim ball three times a day for ten minutes a time. The Vilim Ball is a small circle-shaped device that produces vibrating sensations that can reduce essential hand tremors by up to 50%, resulting in up to four hours of relief from essential hand tremors, allowing individuals relief, time and the ability to perform daily life tasks without consistent tremors. It can be purchased at www.vilimed.com
- I also notice that in cold weather my tremor gets worse.
- There is a website that I use called www.novitatech.com.au NovitaTech combines creative thinking and technology to enhance human capability. I have bought a lot of assisted technology devices from them which has made my life so much simpler!

For example:

- Slip on sneakers that do not require me to bend down or do up shoelaces
- Linen shirts with magnets for buttons
- Automatic jar openers
- Hand steady drinking mug
- Stabilizing soup spoon

3. Restleg Legs

My nights can be a living hell. Just when you think Parkinson's has taken enough from you, Restless Legs Syndrome creeps in like a sadistic torturer. It's not enough that your dreams become a battlefield – no, your own legs have to betray you too.

The sensations – they're not just uncomfortable, they're maddening. It's like ants crawling under your skin, like your bones are on fire. The urge to move isn't a gentle nudge, it's a primal scream from deep within your body. You pace the dark, silent house like a caged animal, desperate for even a moment's relief.

The pain. Oh, the pain. It rips through you, leaving you a sobbing mess at 3 AM, feeling utterly alone and broken. You want to claw your own skin off just to make it stop. It's not just physical – it's soul-crushing, stealing whatever scraps of normalcy or dignity you've managed to hold onto.

In those bleak hours, it feels like your body is waging war against your very existence. Haven't you suffered enough? Haven't you lost enough sleep, enough peace, enough of yourself to this disease?

Your husband's hands in the darkness are a lifeline, the only thing anchoring you to sanity some nights. His massages aren't just touching muscle and bone – they're touching your battered spirit, reminding you that you're still loved, still human, even when your own body seems intent on destroying you.

This is the hidden torment of Parkinson's. The relentless, grinding assault that happens behind closed doors, that steals your rest and leaves you facing each new day already exhausted and defeated. It's a battle you never asked for, against an enemy you can't see or reason with. Yet, somehow, you keep fighting, night after endless night.

Suggested solutions

- I am fortunate to have an electric bed with a massage function so now I put that on during the night
- I rub magnesium on my legs and the bottom of my feet (which was kindly suggested by one of my You Tube followers)
- My electric blanket goes on when it gets really bad
- I have a massage band that I fit around my thigh which I use to stimulate circulation
- I now sleep with satin sheets. It is so much easier to roll over in the middle of the night and to get out of bed!
- I also take slow releasing paracetamol which does the job!

4. Toilet Issues

Alright, buckle up buttercups, because I'm about to take you on a wild ride through the most mortifying yet hilarious chapter of my Parkinson's journey. This story is so embarrassing, it practically deserves its own Netflix special. But hey, if we can't laugh at ourselves, what's the point, right?

I was in Melbourne, the fashion capital of Australia, dressed to the nines. We're talking slacks, a silky blouse and heels that made my feet cry but my legs look fabulous. My hair was coiffed to perfection, and my makeup? Let's just say I could've walked straight onto a magazine cover. (okay, that's a stretch!) I was ready for a day of self-love and retail therapy, armed with my credit card and a burning desire to own every shiny thing I laid my eyes on.

Now, for us Parkinson's warriors, constipation is usually our unwelcome sidekick. It's like having a clingy friend who just won't take the hint and leave. So when I felt the urge to go, I was actually excited. Yes, you read that right - I was thrilled about poop. That's what Parkinson's does to you, folks! It turns normal bodily functions into cause for celebration. "Alert the media! She's going to poop!"

I strutted into this fancy-schmancy mall - we're talking marble floors so shiny you could see your reflection, chandeliers that would make any pop star want to swing from them and shop windows displaying clothes with price tags that made my credit card whimper in fear. It was like the Buckingham Palace of shopping centres and I was ready to be crowned Queen of Retail.

That's when it happened. My bowels, those treacherous organs, decided to stage a coup. There was no warning, no time to find a bathroom, just a sudden, urgent need to evacuate the premises, if you know what I mean.

There I was, in my loose slacks (thank goodness for small mercies), when suddenly - oh, the humanity! - I watched in horror as a log rolled out onto the floor. Yes, an actual log. On marble. In public. It was like watching a train wreck in slow motion, except the train was my dignity and the wreck was... well, you get the picture.

But wait, there's more! Because apparently, my body decided that one embarrassing incident wasn't enough. What followed was a tsunami of... let's just say it rhymes with 'diarrhea' and leave it at that. There I was, standing in a puddle of my own making, in the middle of this luxurious mall, wondering if I could pass this off as performance art.

Did I mention I couldn't find a bathroom? Oh, and when I finally did, there was no toilet paper. Because of course there wasn't! At this point, I was half-naked, wrapped in my daughter's tiny blazer that I'd fortunately been carrying. It barely covered my essentials!

I had to do the world's most unglamorous catwalk between bathrooms, playing a game of 'run, wet, wash, repeat'. Picture a penguin with its legs tied together, trying to waddle gracefully across an ice rink. That was me, except less graceful and more... moist.

The grand finale? Having to shop for new clothes in designer stores, with one thigh exposed like I was some sort of accidental burlesque dancer. There I was, sheepishly asking sales assistants if they had anything in the 'I just had an accident' collection. Their faces were a mix of horror, pity and 'please don't touch anything'.

I finally found a store that took pity on me and let me change in their dressing room. As I emerged in my new, overpriced outfit, I couldn't help but laugh. There I was, looking like a million bucks (or at least the couple hundred I'd just spent), with a story that was priceless.

So there you have it, folks. My dignity took a vacation that day, but my sense of humour? It's still going strong. Because if Parkinson's thinks it can embarrass me into submission, it's got another thing coming. I'm here, I'm bare (sometimes unintentionally) and I'm not going anywhere!

And let me tell you, dear readers, this experience taught me a few valuable lessons:

   1. Always, ALWAYS carry spare clothes and toilet paper. And maybe a hazmat suit.

   2. Marble floors are not your friend when you're having a 'movement' issue.

   3. Laughter truly is the best medicine, especially when combined with actual medicine.

4. Parkinson's might control my body sometimes, but it will never control my spirit or my ability to find humour in the absurd.

So next time you're having a bad day, just remember: at least you didn't poop in a fancy mall in Melbourne. If you did... well, welcome to the club! We meet on Thursdays, bring your own wet wipes.

Suggested solutions

- Diet is extremely important, make sure you are getting enough fibre (and not too much too!)
- Extremely important that this symptom is discussed at length with your care team

5. Dystonia

Living with dystonia as part of my Parkinson's has been a strange and sometimes unsettling journey. It crept up on me slowly at first, a whisper of something not quite right in my left foot. I remember the first time I noticed it - a slight curling of my toes that I couldn't quite control. It was as if my foot had developed a mind of its own, rebelling against my attempts to keep it flat and steady.

As time went on, this odd sensation evolved into something more pronounced. My foot began to arch dramatically, like a dancer's, but without any of the grace or intention. It was frustrating and, at times, embarrassing. I'd catch myself walking differently, trying to compensate for this unwelcome change in my body.

The moments when I become most aware of my dystonia are often when I'm trying to relax. There's a cruel irony in sitting down to watch TV or settling in for a drive, only to feel my foot start to claw and curl. It's as if my body is reminding me that even in stillness, Parkinson's is always there, always active.

I've heard other people with Parkinson's talk about the pain that comes with their dystonia and I feel a mix of guilt and relief that I've been spared that particular torment. But even without pain, there's an emotional weight to carrying this symptom. It's a constant reminder of how Parkinson's is changing me, altering even the simplest aspects of my physical existence.

There are days when I feel like a stranger in my own body. I find myself staring at my left foot, willing it to behave, to lie flat and still like its partner. Sometimes, in quieter moments, I feel a wave of sadness wash over me. This isn't how I imagined my body would betray me as I aged.

Yet, there's also a part of me that's grown stronger through this experience. I've become more attuned to my body, more aware of its quirks and needs. I've learned to adapt, to find new ways of moving and being that accommodate this changed part of me. In that adaptation, I've found a resilience I didn't know I possessed.

Living with dystonia, with Parkinson's, is a daily exercise in patience and self-compassion. It's taught me to appreciate the good days, to be gentle with myself on the harder ones and to find humour where I can in the odd twists and turns my body takes. It's not the journey I would have chosen, but it's mine and I'm determined to walk it - curled toes and all - with as much grace as I can muster.

Suggested solutions

- I work very hard to change the "habitual loop" in my brain by being aware when my foot 'curls' and then press it flat
- It is worth seeing a podiatrist. I saw a Biomechanical Podiatrist who conducted a thorough assessment to examine the way my lower limbs work, which enabled them to check for potential abnormalities and possible causes of foot pain, as well as pain in the ankle, knee and back if present

The day I realised I had to say goodbye to my beloved high heels was a tough one. It felt like I was giving up a part of my identity, another small sacrifice to Parkinson's. But as I've learned to navigate life with dystonia, I've come to appreciate the importance of proper footwear more than I ever thought possible.

Now, my shoe choices revolve around comfort and stability rather than style. Solid sneakers have become my new best friends. The way they cradle my foot, providing support for my unpredictable arch, has been a game-changer. It's amazing how much difference the right shoe can make - not just in managing the dystonia, but in my overall confidence when walking.

I've had to completely overhaul my wardrobe to match my new footwear needs. No more delicate strappy sandals or sleek pumps. Instead, I'm always on the lookout for shoes that offer a good balance of support and flexibility. It's been a journey of trial and error, finding brands and styles that work best with my curling toes and arching foot.

There are days when I miss the elegance of dressing up in heels, especially for special occasions. But I've come to realise that feeling secure on my feet, reducing the risk of falls and minimising discomfort are far more important than any fashion statement.

This shift in footwear has become a visible reminder of how I'm adapting to life with Parkinson's. It's a small thing, really, in the grand scheme of this condition. But it's these small adaptations that add up, helping me navigate each day with a bit more ease and a lot more stability.

6. Acting out my dreams

Normally, the body is paralyzed during REM sleep, which is when dreams occur. In certain conditions, such as Parkinson's, the "off" switch doesn't work, so then a person might "act out" dreams without knowledge of doing so

"Folks, gather 'round for the wildest bedtime story you've ever heard. Welcome to my nightly adventures with Parkinson's, where sleep is optional and chaos is guaranteed!"

First up, we have the 'Potty-Mouth Puppet Show'. Apparently, when I'm asleep, I turn into a sailor with a vocabulary that would make Gordon Ramsay blush. My poor husband gets a front-row seat to this R-rated monologue every night. I wake up none the wiser, while he's wondering if he should wash my mouth out with soap. Maybe I should start a late-night comedy show - 'Parkinson's After Dark: Where the Jokes Are Involuntary and Always Dirty!'

But wait, there's more! We've also got 'The Midnight Wrestler'. In this thrilling event, I transform into a WWE superstar, complete with punches, kicks and probably a mean elbow drop. My husband, bless his heart, is the unwilling opponent in this match. He signed up for 'in sickness and in health', not 'in UFC and in bruises'. I'm thinking of getting him a referee whistle for Christmas.

Now, for the main event: 'The Incredible Hulk Meets Interior Designer'. Picture this: It's 3 AM and my husband wakes up to find me, all 172cm of me, casually moving a full length mirror that I can't budge when I'm awake. Talk about your unexpected superpowers! I'm like a bizarre superhero - 'By day, a normal woman with Parkinson's. By night, MIRROR MOVER!' Maybe I should start a midnight moving company. Slogan: 'We only work when we're asleep, but boy, do we work!'

The best part? I remember none of this. It's like Vegas, baby - what happens in dream-land, stays in dream-land. Except, you know, for the evidence. The stories and the bruises!

My poor daughter, bless her, gets roped into these shenanigans too. Nothing says 'family bonding' quite like being woken up at 3 AM to confirm that no, she didn't move a 200-pound mirror for funsies. I'm pretty sure this isn't what the parenting books meant by 'creating lasting memories'.

You'd think after all this, we'd opt for separate bedrooms. But nope! We're sticking together like glue, just in case I attempt to sleepwalk out the window if left unsupervised. It's romance, Parkinson's style - where 'I've got your back' means 'I'm literally holding you back from rearranging the furniture in your sleep'.

So here's to another night of adventure! Will I curse like a drunken pirate? Punch like Mike Tyson? Redecorate like a caffeinated Netflix host? Who knows! It's like a box of chocolates, except instead of chocolates, it's a mix of terror, confusion and unintentional comedy.

Parkinson's might think it's the star of this show, but I've got news for it - I'm the real headliner here. So bring it on, you neurological nightmare! I've got puns, I've got guts and I've got a husband who's probably seriously considering wearing shin pads to bed.

Sweet dreams, everyone! Remember, if you hear screaming, swearing, or the sound of furniture moving in the middle of the night... Well, it's probably just me, living my best life. Or worse. It's hard to tell sometimes!"

Suggested solutions

- Apparently taking Melatonin at night helps but to be honest it hasn't worked for me
- There is a band that you can buy to wear around your foot which vibrates when you get up and put your full weight on it. I haven't tried this because of my toilet issues during the night but hey.... That little ripper is still to come!
- I am currently researching a device to monitor my night time movements and to alert my family if I move from the bed and potentially risk unsafe behaviours

Other than that I suggest you don't invite me to sleep at your house, unless of course you need furniture moved!

7. Apathy

"Apathy. It's a simple word, just six letters long, but it carries a weight heavier than most can imagine. As someone living with Parkinson's Disease, I've come to know this weight intimately and it's a burden that crushes not just the spirit, but the very essence of who I am.

Before apathy crept into my life, I was a force of nature. Determination ran through my veins, ambition fueled my days, and dreams lit up my nights. I had goals, both big and small, that kept me moving forward. I cherished my relationships, thrived on social interactions and found joy in the simplest of activities. Even when first faced with the challenges of

Parkinson's, I held onto that spark, that zest for life that defined me.

I had battled depression before, so I thought I knew the depths of emotional struggle. The sadness, the hopelessness, the dark cloud that seems to follow you everywhere - these were familiar foes. But apathy? It opened up a chasm I never knew existed, a void so vast and empty it swallowed everything I thought I was.

It came silently, insidiously. There was no dramatic shift, no sudden change. Instead, it was a slow erosion of my will, my desires, my very self. By the time my Parkinson's counsellor pointed it out, it had already taken root deep within me. The relisation was like a punch to the gut – how could I not have noticed this fundamental shift in my being?

This isn't depression. Depression, at least, is feeling something even if it's pain or sadness. Apathy is the absence of feeling, the void where emotion should be. It's not "I can't" or "I won't" – it's "I don't care." That, perhaps, is the cruellest twist of all. It's as if someone has drained all the colour from your world, leaving you in a grayscale existence where nothing truly matters.

My once vibrant life began to fade like an old photograph. Exercise, once a cornerstone of my routine and a vital part of managing my Parkinson's symptoms, became a distant memory. The trainers at the gym, who used to greet me with encouraging smiles, now probably wondered if I'd fallen off the face of the earth. My running shoes gathered dust in the corner, silent reminders of the person I used to be.

My social circle, previously bustling with energy and laughter, fell silent. Invitations to gatherings went unanswered, not because I didn't want to go, but because I couldn't muster the energy to care either way. Friends' concerned messages piled up in my inbox, each one a pang of guilt that I couldn't even fully feel.

Communication dwindled to nothing. Calls went straight to voicemail, texts remained unread. It wasn't a conscious decision to isolate myself - it was the absence of any decision at all. The thought of reaching out, of engaging, felt as monumental as climbing Everest and as pointless as trying to empty the ocean with a teaspoon.

It was as if I had simply... stopped. Stopped trying, stopped caring, stopped living. The hobbies that once brought me joy now lay abandoned. Books remained unread, my garden overgrown. The world continued to spin, but I had stepped off, watching it all pass by with detached indifference.

The most heartbreaking part? I couldn't even bring myself to care about not caring. It was a new low, a rock bottom with a trap door. Parkinson's had won and I couldn't even muster the energy to wave the white flag of surrender. There was no fight left in me, no desire to push back against this invisible force that had hollowed me out.

This is the face of apathy – a blank stare, a shrug, a life lived in grayscale. It's the thief that steals not just your joy, but your sadness too, leaving nothing but a vast, echoing emptiness. It's waking up each morning and feeling no difference between a new day and the end of the world. It's watching your own life slip away and feeling nothing more than a vague, distant acknowledgment of the fact.

To my friends, my family, my loved ones – I'd see the pain in their eyes, the confusion, the hurt. I know they were reaching out, trying to pull me back from this abyss. I hear your voices, but they're muffled, as if I'm underwater. I want to respond, to reach back, but my arms feel leaden, my voice trapped. I see the worry lines deepening on your faces, the frustration in your gestures and I know I'm the cause. But even that knowledge fails to penetrate the thick fog of apathy that surrounds me.

I remember the person I used to be - the one who planned adventures, who laughed easily, who cared deeply. That person feels like a stranger now, a character in a story I once read but can barely recall. There are moments when I catch a glimpse of her in the mirror and for a split second, I feel a flicker of... something. Longing? Regret? But before I can grasp it, it's gone, swallowed by the void.

This is the cruel dichotomy of apathy – intellectually knowing you should care, but emotionally unable to do so. It's a prison where you're both the inmate and the warden, but you've lost the key and can't bring yourself to look for it. You're trapped in a paradox of your own making, aware of the problem but incapable of mustering the will to solve it.

The world continues to turn. Seasons change, holidays come and go, life events unfold. But it all happens at a distance, as if I'm watching it on a television with the volume turned down. Birthdays pass uncelebrated, anniversaries unmarked. The milestones that once brought excitement or anticipation now elicit nothing more than a shrug.

Yet, somewhere deep inside, buried under layers of apathy and indifference, there's a tiny spark that refuses to be extinguished completely. It's faint, barely perceptible, but it's there. Perhaps it's the last remnant of the person I used to be, or maybe it's the seed of the person I could become. Either way, its presence is both a comfort and a torment - a reminder that feeling is possible, even if it seems unreachable.

So there I stood, or perhaps 'existed' is a better word. A shadow of my former self, wrestling with an opponent I never saw coming. Maybe, just maybe, acknowledging this beast is the first step towards reclaiming the life it stole from me.

To anyone else drowning in this sea of apathy – you're not alone. Your feelings, or lack thereof, are valid. This is not your fault. It's not a choice you made or a weakness in your character. It's a symptom, just like tremors or stiffness, but one that attacks the very core of who you are.

Even if you can't see it right now, you are worth fighting for. We are worth fighting for. There is a world of colour waiting for us beyond this gray fog, a symphony of emotions ready to play once we find our way back. It won't be easy and there will be days when it seems impossible. But we owe it to ourselves, and to those who love us, to keep trying.

Because somewhere inside us, buried deep beneath the apathy, is the person we used to be. That person is still worth saving.

Suggested solutions

- I encourage you to speak with a trained counsellor, hopefully one specialising in Parkinson's.
- Once I understood what apathy was and how I was being impacted, I wrote down a list of what was important to me and started taking small steps towards that.
- Exercise is critical in pulling yourself out of apathy. It gives you back a sense of control as well as blood flow increases, your brain is exposed to more oxygen and nutrients. Exercise also induces the release of beneficial proteins in the brain. These nourishing proteins keep brain cells (also known as neurons) healthy and promote the growth of new neurons. Neurons are the working building blocks of the brain.

8. Dyskinesias - International Travel

Dyskinesias are involuntary, erratic, writhing movements of the face, arms, legs or trunk. They are often fluid and dance-like, but they may also cause rapid jerking or slow and extended muscle spasms.

I never thought my love for travel would become a race against time. But here I am, frantically ticking off bucket list destinations before my body decides to ground me permanently. Parkinson's, you cruel thief of dreams.

Our recent flight from Australia to Kuala Lumpur... I can still feel the shame burning my cheeks. It started in the airport, my body betraying me before we even boarded. I was jerking like a marionette with a sadistic puppeteer, my limbs flailing in a grotesque dance. My darling husband, bless him, kept whispering, "Breathe, Lisa, breathe." But how do you breathe when your body's rebelling and everyone's staring?

For six hours on that plane, I dared to hope. Maybe, just maybe, I'd make it through unscathed. Fool's hope.

When dyskinesia hit, it hit hard. My neck turned to jelly, my head lolling like a newborn's. Then my torso, my arms - it was like my body was trying to disassemble itself mid-flight. The pain... How do I even describe it? It was as if every nerve ending was screaming in protest.

But the physical agony? That was nothing compared to the emotional torment. I sobbed - deep, guttural sobs that came from a place of utter despair and humiliation. There I was, a grown woman, unable to control my own body, making a spectacle of myself in a metal tube hurtling through the sky.

Then I saw my husband's face. Oh, that look in his eyes - it haunts me still. Worry, fear, helplessness - all swirling in those eyes I've loved for so long. At that moment, I felt my heart shatter. This disease isn't just stealing from me; it's robbing him too. Robbing us of the golden years we'd dreamed of, replacing them with... this.

Yet, here's the kicker - I'm not ready to give up. Call it stubbornness or madness but I refuse to let Parkinson's clip my wings just yet. Yes, each trip is a gamble now. Yes, the day may come when long-haul flights are a distant memory. But until then? I'll keep packing my bags, keep exploring this beautiful world, keep making memories with the man who holds my hand through every shake and tremor.

So to Parkinson's, I say: You may slow me down, you may make me stumble, but you will not stop me. Not yet. I've got too much world to see, too much life to live. To my fellow travellers wrestling with chronic illness: We might not be able to control our bodies, but we can control our spirits. Let's keep exploring, keep adventuring, keep living - wobbles, jerks and all. Our journeys may look different now, but they're still beautiful.

Suggested solutions

- I now save that little bit longer and fly Premium Economy. It is way cheaper than Business Class but gives you so much more room than Economy
- I take my disabled pass EVERYWHERE when I travel. This allows me to check-in at priority lanes (so I do not have to queue), I board the plane first (which eliminates me holding everyone up), It also allows me priority access at immigration. Standing in long lines is not my friend!
- I try to fly overnight so that I can take a sleeping tablet
- Really important to stay on time when your medication is due!

MY MESSAGE TO THOSE WHO ARE IN GOOD HEALTH

Ladies and gentlemen, my name is Lisa Bradbury and I write to you today as a woman living with a ticking time bomb inside my own body. I have Parkinson's Disease - a ruthless, incurable condition that is slowly robbing me of control over my own flesh and bones. The future that lies ahead of me is not just unpleasant; it's a nightmare I wouldn't wish upon my worst enemy.

My left hand - my dominant hand. It is trembling? It's not a friendly wave; it's the visible mark of my daily battle. But don't pity me. Instead, let this tremor serve as a stark reminder of how quickly life can change.

You know, it's funny how life throws curveballs at you. Before my diagnosis, I was always in control. I prided myself on my steady hands - whether I was typing up reports, preparing presentations, or even just enjoying a cup of coffee. Now, that same hand betrays me daily. But here's the kicker - this very symptom has become my unexpected social lubricant. I've made more accidental friends from people thinking I'm waving at them than I ever did before!

Now, brace yourselves as I plunge you into a chilling thought experiment. Imagine this: would you rather be born with a disability, or live half your life in blissful health only to have it ripped away from you in your prime? It's not just a hypothetical question for me - it's my brutal reality.

The truth is, in our world today, the specter of disease looms larger than ever. Take Parkinson's - the rate of diagnoses have skyrocketed by a staggering 81% since the turn of the millennium. It's a tidal wave of neurological devastation, striking down people younger and younger each year. I was 48 when I was diagnosed. Just think about that for a moment - 48. I was in the prime of my life, at the peak of my career, with teenage children who still needed me to be strong and active.

I've lived on both sides of this cruel divide - the blissful ignorance of health and the harsh awakening of chronic illness. Let me tell you, the transformation is earth-shattering. It's not just your body that changes; your entire world view gets turned upside down every single day.

Before my diagnosis, I was a force to be reckoned with in the corporate world. I climbed the ladder, shattered glass ceilings and thought I was invincible. Little did I know that just months later, I'd be sitting in a doctor's office, hearing words that would change my life forever.

Today, I feel like a living memento - a reminder of mortality with one foot already in the grave. Parkinson's is my constant companion, a relentless foe that I grapple with every waking moment. The regret of not having lived life to its fullest when I had the chance haunts me like a ghost.

But I'm not here to simply share my woes. No, I'm here to shake you awake, to jolt you out of your complacency before it's too late. The life you take for granted today could be gone tomorrow. So listen closely as I share the hard-earned wisdom I've gained from dancing with death.

First and foremost, engrave this truth into your hearts: you are not immortal. Each heartbeat brings you closer to your last. Ask yourself, are you squandering your precious time away, or are you squeezing every drop of joy and meaning from each moment? Life isn't just short - it's a fleeting whisper in the wind. Grab it before it slips through your fingers!

How many times have you heard people say "I'll travel the world when I retire," or. "I'll spend more time with my family once this big project is over." Now, those dreams seem like cruel jokes to me. Don't make my mistakes. Start living now.

Your body is not just a vessel; it's the only home you'll ever truly have. Every morsel of food, every drop of drink is either medicine or poison. I love this - "Toxicity brings toxins." It isn't just a catchy phrase - it's a dire warning. Are you nourishing your temple or desecrating it?

I'll admit, I used to fuel my busy lifestyle with quick, processed foods and too much caffeine. I thought I was invincible. Now, I'd give anything to go back and make healthier choices. Every bite matters, folks. Choose wisely.

Stress isn't just uncomfortable - it's a silent assassin. It creeps into your body, poisoning your cells, fraying your nerves. In fact, it is fast becoming the underlying issue for many debilitating illnesses. Meditation, therefore, isn't a luxury; it's a lifeline. Learn to meditate! Even five minutes a day can mean the difference between you having a breakdown and you building resilience.

I remember scoffing at the idea of meditation. "I don't have time for that new-age nonsense," I'd say. Oh, how wrong I was. Now, those few minutes of peace each day are my sanctuary, my lifeline. Give your brain the respite it desperately needs before it's too late because it is only when we meditate, that our mind stops so that it can not only rest but repair itself!

Move it or lose it - that's not just a fitness slogan, it's a prophecy. I was once an Australian gymnast, my body a finely-tuned machine. Now, there are days when I feel like a rusted tin man, creaking and groaning with every movement. Don't wait until your body betrays you. Move, stretch, challenge yourself every single day. Your future self will thank you - or curse you if you don't. No need to run marathons or pump iron like the rock. Gentle, consistent movement is enough!

Some days for me, just getting out of bed is a victory. But I keep moving, because I know that every step, every stretch, is a battle won against this disease.

Wake up! Your job won't comfort you on your deathbed. I was once a corporate warrior, my phone an extension of my arm. But let me tell you a harsh truth - your bosses won't be shedding tears at your funeral. If you're a leader, your actions echo through your entire team. Are you setting an example of work-life balance, or are you propagating a culture of burnout? Do you leave loudly to take your kids to tennis practice once a week because let me tell you, the years that you are missing with your children you will not get back!

When I look back, I'm horrified at the "urgent meeting" or "conference call" that replaced time with my family. Now, I'd trade all my career success for those lost moments. Don't make my mistakes.

Here's a radical idea that might just save your life: love yourself fiercely. More than your spouse, more than your children, more than anyone. It's not selfish - it's survival. If you can't put your own oxygen mask on first, you'll be no good to anyone else when the plane goes down. Even by implementing some changes after this talk is an act of self-love and compassion!

For years, I put everyone else first - my kids, my spouse, my job. I thought that's what a good person does. But in neglecting myself, I was slowly dying inside. Now, I know better. Self-love isn't selfish; it's essential.

Finally, embrace the marvel of neuroplasticity. Your brain is not set in stone - it's a dynamic, ever-changing miracle. You have the power to rewire your own mind, to forge new neural pathways and possibilities. Change the way you think, dance like nobody's watching and allow your brain to form new connections to keep it strong! I'm betting my life on this power, fighting to slow down and even reverse my Parkinson's symptoms.

Every day, I challenge my brain in new ways. I learn new words, try new hobbies, force my trembling hands to attempt intricate tasks. It's hard, it's frustrating, but it's also empowering. I'm not just accepting my fate; I'm fighting back, rewiring my brain one synapse at a time.

If only we truly understood the capabilities of our brain! Your brain believes every word that you tell it. So what story are you feeding it? One of limitation and fear, or one of boundless potential?

You are the architect of your own destiny. Every thought, every action is either reinforcing old patterns or blazing new trails. Are you just going through the motions, or are you consciously crafting the life and mind you desire?

I implore you - don't wait for a diagnosis to start living. Don't wait for your body to fail you before you start appreciating it. Implement these life-changing practices now, today, this very moment.

Carry with you this final, burning truth: growing old with health and vitality is not a right - it's a precious, precious privilege. One that's denied to far too many of us. What is it going to take for you to change your life?

Will you heed this wake-up call? Or will you slumber on, only to be rudely awakened when it's far too late? The choice, my friends, is yours. Choose wisely, for your very life depends on it.

Remember, every moment is a gift. Every breath is an opportunity. Don't squander them. Live fully, love fiercely and never, ever take your health for granted. Because trust me, when it's gone, you'll realise it was the greatest wealth you ever had.

Now go out there and write a better one for yourselves. Your future self is counting on you.

About Lisa Bradbury

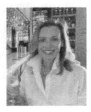

Lisa's journey to becoming an advocate for integrative health and wellness began long before her own diagnosis. Growing up with a sister diagnosed with Muscular Dystrophy, she gained early insights into the challenges of chronic illness and the resilience it demands.

A natural athlete, Lisa's dedication and talent led her to represent Australia in Rhythmic Gymnastics at the Australian Institute of Sport at just 11 years old. This early experience instilled in her a deep understanding of the body's potential and the power of disciplined practice.

Her compassionate nature shone through in her corporate career, where she won the title of Miss NSW Fundraiser in 1999, raising money for children with Cerebral Palsy. But it was becoming a mother to Zachary and Jamieson at 30 that Lisa considers her greatest reward and accomplishment.

Life took an unexpected turn when Lisa was diagnosed with Parkinson's at age 48. Rather than letting this define her limitations, she saw it as a call to action. Determined to understand her condition and explore all possible avenues for wellness, Lisa embarked on a journey of education and personal growth.

She became a certified Mind-Body Practitioner, opening her world to alternative methods of healing. Her quest for knowledge didn't stop there. Lisa went on to become a Life Coach specializing in Health and Wellbeing, and later an Ageless Grace Educator, diving deep into the science of neuroplasticity.

Today, Lisa is a living example of the power of positive thinking and the strength of the human spirit. Through her YouTube channel, "Positively Parkinson's," she shares her insights and inspires others facing similar challenges.

This book represents Lisa's latest endeavor to spread hope and empower others. It's a testament to her belief that with the right mindset, knowledge, and approach, anything is possible – even in the face of a life-altering diagnosis.

When she's not writing, or creating content for her channel, Lisa can be found practicing Ageless Grace exercises, exploring new holistic wellness techniques, and cherishing time with her family. She continues to approach life with the same grace, determination, and positive spirit that has carried her from the gymnastics mat to becoming a beacon of hope for those navigating chronic illness.

This is what other people have to say about this book

"Lisa is an exceptional human and this book is a testament of her intellect, knowledge, humour and courage. So raw in places that you cringe but so honestly and beautifully written you feel like you're on her journey. I don't have Parkinson's but have suffered for years with depression and anxiety. The tools, links and practical advice I found personally invaluable. I have no doubt Lisa will cure her Parkinson's, if her mindset and attitude is any to go by. This book is going to help millions. A bloody good read. "

Debra Ellen

Melbourne, Australia

"Thank goodness Lisa has a lot to say about her journey. Her real and raw story is hugely insightful for carers to also fully understand every day life for those with Parkinson's Disease. The treatment and lifestyle options researched for this book showcase an array of possibilities giving the reader solid options to consider.
Stay fierce."

Debbie Fisher

Canberra, Australia (Carer)

"I'm so proud of my wife to push through Parkinson's head winds and keep smiling and finding work arounds every day. This book represent her soul, it brings wings to her mind and flight to her imaginations"

Real and raw as she would say with comical overlay of our everyday life ."

Simon Bradbury

Adelaide, Australia (Husband)

Made in United States
Orlando, FL
05 June 2025